Handbook of
Targeted Cancer Therapy and Immunotherapy
Breast Cancer

Handbook of
Targeted Cancer Therapy and Immunotherapy
Breast Cancer

Editors

Senthil Damodaran, MD, PhD

Assistant Professor
Division of Cancer Medicine
Department of Breast Medical Oncology
Department of Investigational Cancer Therapeutics
The University of Texas MD Anderson Cancer Center
Houston, Texas

Debu Tripathy, MD

Professor and Chair
Department of Breast Medical Oncology
The University of Texas MD Anderson Cancer Center
Houston, Texas

Series Editors

Daniel D. Karp, MD

Professor of Medicine
Department of Investigational Cancer Therapeutics
Principal Investigator of the MD Anderson Clinical & Translational Science Award (CTSA)
The University of Texas MD Anderson Cancer Center
Houston, Texas

Gerald S. Falchook, MD, MS

Director
Drug Development Unit
Sarah Cannon Research Institute at HealthONE
Presbyterian/St. Luke's Medical Center
Denver, Colorado

JoAnn D. Lim, PharmD, BCOP

Clinical Pharmacy Specialist, Phase I
Division of Pharmacy
Department of Investigational Cancer Therapeutics
The University of Texas MD Anderson Cancer Center
Houston, Texas

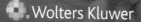

Wolters Kluwer

Philadelphia · Baltimore · New York · London
Buenos Aires · Hong Kong · Sydney · Tokyo

Acquisitions Editor: Nicole Dernoski
Development Editor: Eric McDermott
Editorial Coordinator: Priyanka Alagar
Marketing Manager: Kirsten Watrud
Production Project Manager: Catherine Ott
Manager of Graphic Arts and Design: Stephen Druding
Manufacturing Coordinator: Beth Welsh
Prepress Vendor: S4Carlisle Publishing Services

9 8 7 6 5 4 3 2 1

Printed in Mexico

Library of Congress Cataloging-in-Publication Data

ISBN-13: 978-1-9751-8456-8

Cataloging in Publication data available on request from publisher.

shop.lww.com

QUADM08 22

Contributors

Kavitha Balaji, PhD
AstraZeneca

Sarah Baldwin, RN, ANP-BC, BSN, MSN
The University of Texas MD Anderson Cancer Center

Tamara G. Barnes, RN, MSN, CNS, AOCNS
The University of Texas MD Anderson Cancer Center

Laura Beatty, PA-C
The University of Texas MD Anderson Cancer Center

Lindsay Gaido Bramwell, MSN, RN, ACNS-BC
Flatiron Health

Sara Bresser, MPAS, PA-C
The University of Texas MD Anderson Cancer Center

Amanda Brink, DNP, APRN, FNP-BC, AOCNP
The University of Texas MD Anderson Cancer Center

Isabel Cepeda, MSN, RN, AGN-P
The University of Texas MD Anderson Cancer Center

Hui Chen, MD, PhD
The University of Texas MD Anderson Cancer Center

Niamh Coleman, MD, PhD
The University of Texas MD Anderson Cancer Center

Senthil Damodaran, MD, PhD
The University of Texas MD Anderson Cancer Center

Ecaterina Dumbrava, MD
The University of Texas MD Anderson Cancer Center

Haven Garber, MD, PhD
The University of Texas MD Anderson Cancer Center

Roman Groisberg, MD
Rutgers Cancer Institute of New Jersey

Toshiaki Iwase, MD, PhD
The University of Texas MD Anderson Cancer Center

Filip Janku, MD, PhD
The University of Texas MD Anderson Cancer Center

Daniel D. Karp, MD
The University of Texas MD Anderson Cancer Center

Ed Kheder, MD
The University of Texas MD Anderson Cancer Center

Holly Kinahan, RN, MSN, NP-C, AOCNP
The University of Texas MD Anderson Cancer Center

Jangsoon Lee, PhD
The University of Texas MD Anderson Cancer Center

JoAnn D. Lim, PharmD, BCOP
The University of Texas MD Anderson
Cancer Center

Kathrina Marcelo-Lewis, PhD
The University of Texas MD Anderson Cancer Center

Hossein Maymani, MD
Rocky Mountain Cancer Centers

Funda Meric-Bernstam, MD
The University of Texas MD Anderson Cancer Center

Sandra Montez, RN
The University of Texas MD Anderson Cancer Center

Shyamm Moorthy, PhD
The University of Texas MD Anderson Cancer Center

Justin Moyers, MD
The University of Texas MD Anderson Cancer Center
University of California, Irvine College of Medicine

Blessie Elizabeth Nelson, MD
The University of Texas MD Anderson Cancer Center

Amy B. Patel, MPAS, PA-C
The University of Texas MD Anderson Cancer Center

Sarina A. Piha-Paul, MD, MS
The University of Texas MD Anderson Cancer Center

Patrick Pilie, MD
The University of Texas MD Anderson Cancer Center

Matthew J. Reilley, MD
University of Virginia

Jordi Rodon-Ahnert, MD, PhD
The University of Texas MD Anderson Cancer Center

Sinchita Roy-Chowdhury, MD, PhD
The University of Texas MD Anderson Cancer Center

Sagar Sardesai, MD, MPH
The Ohio State University

Shiraj Sen, MD, PhD

Ana Stuckett, PhD
The University of Texas MD Anderson Cancer Center

Jasmine Sukumar, MD
The Ohio State University Comprehensive Cancer
Center

Debu Tripathy, MD
The University of Texas MD Anderson Cancer Center

Naoto T. Ueno, MD, PhD, FACP
The University of Texas MD Anderson Cancer Center

Gabriele Urschel, DNP, RN, FNP-C, AOCNP
The University of Texas MD Anderson Cancer Center

Neelima Vidula, MD
Massachusetts General Hospital

Preface

Recent advancements in genomic and proteomic techniques have enabled the clinical development of targeted therapies in breast cancers and other tumor types. Newer targets and therapies are being developed at a rapid pace and it can be quite a daunting task for clinicians and researchers to keep abreast of developments.

Breast cancer laid the foundation for targeted therapy with the discovery of estrogen receptor and endocrine therapy and serves as a prototype for targeted therapies in other tumor types. The goal of this handbook is to provide a concise list of biomarker-driven therapies in breast cancer and make the results of clinical trials of targeted cancer treatments and immunotherapy more easily accessible to clinicians and researchers.

Our objective was to create a handbook that was small enough to fit comfortably into a lab coat pocket so that it may be easily accessible for reference in the clinic. This book was conceived with a broad audience in mind. It is our hope that this book will find use among academic oncologists, community oncologists, researchers, pharmacists, nurses, residents, clinical fellows, midlevel providers, postdoctoral fellows, and other staff who are essential for clinical and translational cancer research. To our knowledge, there is not another book available with the scope of this work in such a concise format for breast cancers.

This book focuses on agents for which clinical data are available, either published or publicly presented at a national meeting. It is possible that clinical trials for which results were not yet available at the time pages were sent for publication may not have been included in this edition. Any exclusion is unintentional, and we apologize in advance to anyone who is surprised or offended to discover that their favorite target/agent was not included. Furthermore, we expect that by the time this work is available for purchase, results of ongoing clinical trials will have become available and could potentially alter the therapeutic landscape of breast cancer.

The book is divided into four core sections. The first section focuses on actionable targets and therapy of interest in breast cancers; the second section focuses on molecular diagnostics and testing that has been created with clinicians in mind; the third section focuses on molecular targets and pathways pertinent to oncology; and the final section describes clinically relevant targeted therapies in breast cancers and solid tumors. We hope that the readers will find the book informative and practical.

Debu Tripathy and Senthil Damodaran

Acknowledgments

We would like to thank the many people who were instrumental in the development of this book. In particular, we would like to express our appreciation to the authors of subsections for their time and willingness to share their knowledge and insights within the pages of this compilation. We would like to thank Thomas Celona, Nicole Dernoski, and other members of Wolters Kluwer Health for their invaluable assistance in the development of this book. We would also like to thank Dr. Falchook and Dr. Karp for their vision and in laying the foundation for this handbook. Above all, we would like to thank our indomitable patients and families for their outstanding contribution to clinical studies without which therapeutic developments in oncology would not have materialized.

Contents

SECTION 3: Molecular Targets and Pathways 105

Ecaterina Dumbrava and Jordi Rodon-Ahnert, Editors

Kavitha Balaji, Ecaterina Dumbrava, Roman Groisberg, Filip Janku, Daniel D. Karp, Ed Kheder, Kathrina Marcelo-Lewis, Hossein Maymani, Sandra Montez, Shyamm Moorthy, Patrick Pilie, Matthew J. Reilley, Jordi Rodon-Ahnert, Shiraj Sen, and Ana Stuckett, Contributors

SECTION 4: Targeted and Immunotherapy Agents 212

JoAnn D. Lim and Justin Moyers, Editors

Sarah Baldwin, Tamara G. Barnes, Laura Beatty, Sara Bresser, Amanda Brink, Isabel Cepeda, Lindsay Gaido Bramwell, Senthil Damodaran, Holly Kinahan, JoAnn D. Lim, Justin Moyers, Amy B. Patel, Debu Tripathy, and Gabriele Urschel, Contributors

Targets of Interest in Breast Cancer

- ADC: antibody–drug conjugate
- AE: adverse event
- Akt: protein kinase B
- AR: androgen receptor
- CBR: clinical benefit rate (CR + PR + SD)
- cfDNA: cell-free DNA
- CI: confidence interval
- CNA: copy number alteration
- CNV: copy number variant
- CPS: combined positive score
- CR: complete response
- CTC: circulating tumor cell
- ctDNA: circulating tumor DNA
- DDT: DNA damage response
- DOR: duration of response
- EGFR: epidermal growth factor receptor
- ER: estrogen receptor
- ET: endocrine therapy
- FDA: U.S. Food and Drug Administration
- FFPE: formalin-fixed paraffin-embedded
- FGFR: fibroblast growth factor receptor
- FISH: fluorescence in situ hybridization
- FNA: fine needle aspiration
- HER2: human epithelial receptor 2
- HR: hazard ratio

- IBTR: ipsilateral breast tumor recurrence
- IHC: immunohistochemistry
- irAE: immune-related adverse event
- ISH: in situ hybridization
- LAR: luminal androgen receptor
- mAb: monoclonal antibody
- MBC: metastatic breast cancer
- mo: month
- MSI: microsatellite instability
- mTOR: mammalian target of rapamycin
- NAT: neoadjuvant therapy
- NGS: next-generation sequencing
- ORR: overall response rate
- OS: overall survival
- PARP: poly (ADP-ribose) polymerase
- PCR: polymerase chain reaction
- PD-1: programmed cell death protein 1
- PD-L1: programmed cell death ligand 1
- PFS: progression-free survival
- PGV: pathogenic germline variant
- PI3K: phosphoinositide 3-kinase
- PIP3: phosphatidylinositol (3,4,5)-trisphosphate
- PR: partial response
- Pts, pt: patients, patient
- ORR: response rate (PR + CR)

- RTK: receptor tyrosine kinase
- RT-PCR: reverse transcriptase polymerase chain reaction
- SD: stable disease
- SERD: selective estrogen receptor downregulator
- SERM: selective estrogen receptor modulator
- SNP: single nucleotide polymorphism
- SNV: single nucleotide variant
- T-DM1: Trastuzumab emtansine
- T-DXd: Trastuzumab deruxtecan
- TACSTD2: Tumor-Associated Calcium Signal Transducer 2
- TCGA: The Cancer Genome Atlas
- TKI: tyrosine kinase inhibitor
- TMB: tumor mutational burden
- TNBC: triple-negative breast cancer
- TRKs: tropomyosin-related kinases
- TROP-2: trophoblast cell-surface antigen 2
- UGT1A1: uridine diphosphate glucuronosyltransferase 1A1
- VAR: variant allele fraction
- VEGFR: vascular endothelial growth factor receptor
- WES: whole-exome sequencing
- WT: wild type

CHAPTER 1

Androgen Receptor

Toshiaki Iwase, Jangsoon Lee, and Naoto T. Ueno

Androgen Receptor

Key points

- Androgen receptor (AR) is frequently expressed in patients with breast cancer (1). However, the threshold for predicting response to inhibitors has not been well established. In previously performed breast cancer clinical trials, 10% and 40% of cutoff by AR IHC expression was applied to ER+/PR+ breast cancer (2,3), 10% and 70% to triple-negative breast cancer (TNBC) (4,5), and 10% to HER2+ breast cancer (6).

- AR expression is associated with favorable prognosis in patients with ER+ breast cancers (7,8)

- The transcriptomic profiling of primary TNBC revealed that high levels of AR IHC expression (≥70%) correlated with the luminal androgen receptor (LAR) gene signature (5)

- Of note, approximately 40% to 50% of LAR tumors harbor *PIK3CA* mutation and some other genomic alterations seen in luminal breast cancer (9,10)

- While further studies are exploring targeting the AR pathway in defined AR-activated cases, this remains investigational and not standard of care

Actionable Target	Abnormality	Prevalence (%)	Clinical Experience with Targeted Agent
AR (ER+)	Overexpression	70%–90% (7,11)	**Enobosarm** (AR agonist) • Phase 2: **AR ≥ 40%**—CBR 80%, median progression-free survival (PFS) 5.47 mo. **AR <40%**—CBR 18%, median PFS 2.72 mo (2). **Enzalutamide** (AR antagonist) • Phase 1/1b with/without endocrine therapy (anastrozole, exemestane, or fulvestrant): CBR at 24 wks—7% (monotherapy) and 9% (with ET) (3) • Phase 2, with exemestane vs. exemestane alone. *No prior ET for MBC*—PFS 11.8 vs. 5.8 mo (HR 0.82, p = 0.363), CBR at 24 wks 39% vs. 29%. PFS 14.0 vs. 5.5 mo (high vs. low AR expression level by mRNA). Prior ET for MBC—PFS 3.6 vs. 3.9 mo (HR 1.02, p =0.92). PFS 4.0 vs. 3.6 mo (high vs. low AR mRNA) (12).

(*continued*)

Actionable Target	Abnormality	Prevalence (%)	Clinical Experience with Targeted Agent
AR (TNBC)	Overexpression	10%–35% (13-16)	**Bicalutamide** (AR antagonist) Phase 2: CBR at 6 mo 19%. PFS 12 wks (13) **Enzalutamide** (AR antagonist) • Phase 2: CBR at 16 wks 25%, CBR at 24 wks 20%. PFS 2.9 mo. OS 12.7 mo (17). • Phase 1b/2, with **taselisib** (PI3K inhibitor): CBR 35.7% (LAR subtype 75.0% vs. non-LAR 12.5%). PFS 3.4 mo (LAR subtype 4.6 vs. non-LAR 2.0 mo) (4). Phase 2, with **paclitaxel.** PCR/RCB-I = 41% (anthracycline-insensitive early TNBC, AR IHC $\geq$ 10%) (5)
AR (HER2+)	Overexpression	60% (8,11)	**Enzalutamide** (AR antagonist) • Phase 2, with **trastuzumab.** CBR at 24 wks 24%. PFS 3.4 mo (metastatic/locally advanced previously treated by anti-HER2 therapy, AR IHC $\geq$ 10%) (6).

CHAPTER 2

BRCA1/2

Neelima Vidula

BRCA1/2

Key points

- *BRCA1/2* are tumor suppressor genes that mediate cellular response to DNA damage. Mutations in the *BRCA1/2* genes can result in the acquisition of more mutations in DNA and ultimately lead to the development of cancer in cells (1,2).

- Germline *BRCA1/2* mutations account for 5% to 10% of breast cancer (3)

- Somatic *BRCA1/2* mutations may be acquired by breast tumors but are thought to be rare. In an analysis of The Cancer Genome Atlas (TCGA), the prevalence of somatic *BRCA1* mutations was observed as 1.55% and the prevalence of somatic *BRCA2* mutations was 1.68%, in primary breast cancer (4). In metastatic disease, the prevalence of pathogenic somatic *BRCA1/2* mutations is higher, estimated at 4% to 6% (5,6).

- Poly (ADP-ribose) polymerase (PARP) inhibitors have been investigated in breast cancer with germline *BRCA1/2* mutations. PARP1 and 2 play an integral role in the cellular response to DNA breaks (7). *In vitro*, *BRCA1/2*-deficient cells are sensitive to PARP inhibition as they cannot repair DNA damage via PARP, leading to cell death (7).

- Two PARP inhibitors, olaparib and talazoparib, are currently approved for the treatment of patients with germline *BRCA1/2* mutations and metastatic hormone receptor + /HER2 − or TNBC, based on randomized trials demonstrating an improvement in PFS with the PARP inhibitors compared to chemotherapy (8,9)

- Olaparib has also been demonstrated to be beneficial as adjuvant therapy, with improved disease-free survival in germline *BRCA1/2* carriers who have early-stage hormone receptor +/HER2 − breast cancer or TNBC (10)

- PARP inhibitors are being investigated in somatic *BRCA1/2* mutant metastatic breast cancer in ongoing clinical trials with olaparib (11) and talazoparib (12)

- *BRCA1/2* reversion mutations, which restore the open reading frame of the *BRCA1/2* gene, may render a PARP inhibitor ineffective, and can be detected in cell-free DNA (6,13)

- Combination studies have explored other combinations with PARP inhibition including immunotherapy for a possible synergistic effect (14,15)

- In addition to germline *BRCA1/2* alterations, olaparib has been shown to have activity in germline *PALB2* and somatic *BRCA1/2* alterations. ORR 82% in germline PALB2 mutations. No responses were observed in *ATM* or *CHEK2* (11).

- There is interest in targeting other members of DDR pathway such as ATM, ATR, WEE1, and RAD51. Early-phase clinical trials target some of these molecules, either as a single agent or in combination with other molecularly targeted agents and immune checkpoint inhibitors (16).

Actionable Target	Abnormality	Prevalence (%)	Clinical Experience with Targeted Agent
BRCA1/2	Mutation/ Deletion	5%–10% (Germline) 4%–6% (Somatic)	**Olaparib (PARP inhibitor) (FDA approved):** • **OlympiAD**, Phase 3, Randomized: PFS 7.0 (Olaparib) vs. 4.2 mo for chemotherapy in germline *BRCA1/2*-mutant, HER2− MBC, HR 0.58, 95% CI 0.43–0.80, $p < 0.001$. ORR 59.9% vs. 28.8%. No OS difference, median OS 19.3 mo (olaparib) vs. 17.1 mo (chemotherapy), HR 0.90, 95% CI 0.66–1.23, $p = 0.513$ (17). • **OLYMPIA**, Phase 3, Randomized: 1 yr of adjuvant olaparib vs. placebo for high-risk, early-stage, germline *BRCA1/2* mutant HER2− breast cancer. 3 yr invasive disease-free survival of 85.9% (olaparib) vs. 77.1% (placebo), HR 0.58, 99.5% CI 0.41–0.82, $p < 0.001$. 3 yr distant disease-free survival of 87.5% (olaparib) vs. 80.4% (placebo), HR 0.57, 99.5% CI 0.39–0.83, $p < 0.001$ (10). • **TBCRC048**. Olaparib in somatic *BRCA1/2*-mutant, HER2− MBC. ORR 50%, CBR 66%, median PFS 6.3 mo (11).

Actionable Target	Abnormality	Prevalence (%)	Clinical Experience with Targeted Agent
			Talazoparib (PARP inhibitor) (FDA approved): • EMBRACA, Phase 3, Randomized. Median PFS 8.6 mo (talazoparib) vs. 5.6 mo (chemotherapy), HR 0.54, 95% CI 0.41–0.71, $p < 0.001$ in *gBRCA1/2*. ORR 63% vs. 27%. Better patient-reported outcomes with talazoparib (9). No improvement in OS. Median OS 19.3 mo with talazoparib vs. 19.5 mo with chemotherapy, HR 0.848, 95% CI 0.670–1.073, $p = 0.17$ (18). • **ABRAZO**, Phase 2: talazoparib in *gBRCA1/2* mutants (Cohort A—response to prior platinum with no progression within 8 wks of last platinum or Cohort B ≥3 platinum-free cytotoxic regimens). ORR 21% and duration of response 5.8 mo (Cohort A); exploratory analysis, longer platinum-free interval was associated with higher ORR in Cohort 1 (0% ORR with interval <8 wks; 47% ORR with interval >6 mo). ORR 37% and DOR 3.8 mo (Cohort B) (19). • **NEOTALA**, Phase 2: neoadjuvant talazoparib (6 mo) in germline *BRCA1/2* carriers. Pathologic complete response rate 53% (20). *(continued)*

Actionable Target	Abnormality	Prevalence (%)	Clinical Experience with Targeted Agent
			Veliparib (PARP inhibitor) • BROCADE3, Phase 3: veliparib with carboplatin and paclitaxel in *BRCA1/2*-mutated, HER2− MBC. Median PFS 14.5 (veliparib/carboplatin/paclitaxel) vs. 12.6 mo (carboplatin/paclitaxel), HR 0.71, 95% CI 0.57–0.88, $p = 0.0016$ (21). **Niraparib (PARP inhibitor)** • TOPACIO, Phase 2: niraparib with pembrolizumab. In *BRCA* mutants, ORR 47%, median PFS 8.3 mo. In *BRCA* WT, ORR 11%, PFS 2.1 mo (22). **Carboplatin** • Phase 3: ORR 68% vs. 33% in *BRCA* mutants (23) • TBCRC009, Phase 2 (carboplatin/cisplatin): ORR 25.6% (overall); ORR 54.5% in germline BRCA carriers (24)

CHAPTER 3

ESR1

Debu Tripathy and Senthil Damodaran

ESR1

Key points

- Estrogen receptors (ERs) exist in two forms, ERα and ERβ, encoded by *ESR1* and *ESR2*, respectively

- ERα is considered a key driver of tumorigenesis in HR+ breast cancers and has served as a basis for the use of endocrine therapy. ERβ is typically expressed in patients with ER− tumors and its role has not been clearly elucidated (1).

- Acquired mutations in ligand-binding domain of *ESR1* are observed in MBC patients exposed to estrogen deprivation with aromatase inhibitor (AI) and are associated with endocrine resistance and poor prognosis (2–5)

- The prevalence of *ESR1* mutations is variable depending on prior exposure to endocrine therapy. *ESR1* mutations are infrequent in primary breast cancers, suggesting clonal selection with exposure (6,7).

- *ESR1* Y537S and D538G are the two most common variants

- *ESR1* mutations tend to be polyclonal and ctDNA analysis has been shown to identify mutations not discernable on tissue sampling (8–11)

- Currently, the most effective therapy for patients harboring *ESR1* mutations is unclear though studies have suggested some of these mutations may exhibit greater sensitivity to fulvestrant (selective estrogen receptor downregulator) and possibly SERMs (selective estrogen receptor modulators) compared to AIs (8,12)

- In SoFEA (Study of Faslodex Versus Exemestane with or without Arimidex) trial, patients with *ESR1* mutations had prolonged PFS with fulvestrant compared with exemestane ($p = 0.02$). No PFS difference was observed in WT *ESR1* (8).

- *ESR1* mutations were observed in 3% of patients at baseline prior to therapy for MBC. In patients with prior exposure to adjuvant AI, the observed prevalence was 7% (13).

- Patients with *ESR1* mutations at baseline have poor PFS compared to patients without (11 vs. 26.7 mo) (13)

- In the BOLERO-2 study (exemestane alone or in combination with everolimus) in HR+ MBC, while *ESR1* mutations were associated with shorter OS compared to WT (32 mo), Y537S mutation (20 mo) was associated with worse outcome compared to D538G (26 mo), suggesting differences in the *ESR1* variants (14)

- Lasofoxifene, a third-generation SERM, has FDA fast-track designation for HR+ MBC patients who harbor *ESR1* mutations and is currently being evaluated in comparison to fulvestrant in the ELAINE study

Actionable Target	Abnormality	Prevalence (%)	Clinical Experience with Targeted Agent
ESR1	Mutation	25–35	<ul><li>Specific variants predict for lack of response to fulvestrant (e.g., Y537S) (14,15)<ul><li>SoFEA trial: In ESR1 mutants, PFS 5.7 for fulvestrant vs. 2.6 mo for exemestane, HR 0.52, 95% CI 0.30–0.92; $p = 0.02$ (8)</li><li>EMBER Phase 1 trial: LY3484356, oral SERD: CBR 48%, irrespective of ESR1 mutation status (16)</li><li>PlasmaMATCH, Phase 2 platform trial: Cohort A, patients with *ESR1* mutations, extended dose fulvestrant: ORR 8%, CBR 12%, DOR 7 mo. Benefit primarily in clonal *ESR1* mutations (17).</li><li>Combined analysis of SoFEA and EFECT trials: In *ESR1* mutants, PFS 2.4 mo with exemestane vs. 3.9 mo (HR 0.59, 95% CI 0.39–0.89; $p = 0.01$) with fulvestrant. In patients without *ESR1* mutation, PFS 4.8 mo (exemestane vs. 4.1 mo with fulvestrant (HR 1.05; 95% CI 0.81–1.37; $p = 0.69$). 1-yr OS 62% vs. 80% ($p = 0.04$). Significant interaction between *ESR1* mutation and treatment ($p = 0.02$) (18).</li><li>Phase 1, Elacestrant (RAD1901), oral SERD. ORR 19.4% in evaluable patients, 33.3% in *ESR1* mutants. CBR 56.5% in *ESR1* mutants (19).</li></ul></li></ul>

CHAPTER 4

PIK3CA

Sagar Sardesai and Jasmine Sukumar

PIK3CA

Key points

- Aberrant activation of the phosphoinositide 3-kinase (PI3K)/protein kinase B (Akt)/ mammalian target of rapamycin (mTOR) pathway is associated with tumor growth, proliferation, and survival (1)

- PI3Ks are grouped into three classes (I–III) according to their substrate preference and sequence homology (2)

- Class I PI3K is a heterodimer with a regulatory and a catalytic subunit. The catalytic subunit, p110, has four isoforms: α, encoded by *PIK3CA*; β, encoded by *PIK3CB*; γ, encoded by *PIK3CG*, and δ, encoded by *PIK3CD* (2).

- Among solid tumors, mutations involving the helical (exon 9) and kinase (exon 20) domains of the p110α isoform are the most common, with mutations in *PIK3CA* observed approximately in 15% of all tumors (3)

- Initial efforts targeting *PIK3CA* mutations have yielded mixed results due to lack of isoform specificity of inhibitors and dose-limiting toxicities

- *PIK3CA* mutations are very heterogenous and their oncogenicity depends on the location of mutation in the gene. Mutations are often observed to coexist with other pathway alterations (e.g., *KRAS, FGFR1*), which can affect clinical response (3,4).

- Double mutations in *PIK3CA* in the same allele (in cis) have been reported to increase sensitivity to PI3Kα inhibitors compared with single-hotspot mutations (5,6). However, in a triplet study of palbociclib, taselisib, and fulvestrant in *PIK3CA*-mutant breast cancers, patients with double mutations had shorter PFS (7).

- *PIK3CA* mutations, while more commonly observed in HR+ breast cancer, are also observed in HER2+ and triple-negative subtypes
- Actionable mutations in nonhelical and nonkinase domains are also less commonly observed (8)
- Additionally, deletions in C2 domain have also been reported in breast cancers (~11%). C2 deletions result in disruption of p85α binding leading to increased p110α activity and sensitivity to PI3Kα inhibitors (9)
- Alpelisib, an alpha-selective PI3K inhibitor, in combination with fulvestrant is FDA approved for *PIK3CA*-mutated, HR+ MBC (10)

Actionable Target	Abnormality	Prevalence (%)	Clinical Experience with Targeted Agent
PIK3CA	Mutation	**ER/PR+:** ~40%	**Everolimus** (mTOR inhibitor) (FDA approved) • **BOLERO-2,** Phase 3, with **exemestane**: ITT-PFS 10.6 vs. 4.1 mo for placebo (11). Benefit maintained regardless of *PIK3CA* alteration. Pts with WT PI3K had greater treatment effect (HR 0.37) vs. mutated PIK3 (HR 0.51). Pts with mutation in Exon 9 mutation (HR 0.26) had greater treatment effect vs. exon 20 (HR 0.56) (12). • Phase 1b in breast and gynecologic malignancies, with **anastrozole**: CBR 27% in pts with PI3K pathway alteration vs. 8% without (13) • **PrE0102,** Phase 2, with **fulvestrant**: PFS 10.3 vs. 5.1 mo with fulvestrant alone (HR 0.61, $p = 0.02$), CBR (63.6% vs. 41.5%; $p = 0.01$) (14) • Phase 2, with **tamoxifen**: CBR 61% vs. 42% for placebo (15) **Alpelisib** (α-selective PI3K inhibitor) (FDA approved) • SOLAR-1, Phase 3, with fulvestrant: PFS 11 vs. 5.7 mo for fulvestrant alone in *PIK3CA* mutants (HR 0.65, $p < 0.001$), PFS 7.4 vs. 5.6 mo (HR 0.85) in non-*PIK3CA* mutated; ORR 6.6% vs. 12.8%, OS 39.3 vs. 31.4 mo (10,16)

Actionable Target	Abnormality	Prevalence (%)	Clinical Experience with Targeted Agent
			• BYLieve, Phase 2 in combination with fulvestrant (Cohort A, after CDK4/6 inhibitor) activity in pts with *PIK3CA* mutation. Median PFS 7.3 mo, 6-mo PFS 54% (17).
			Taselisib (β-sparing PI3K inhibitor)
			• SANDPIPER Phase 3, with fulvestrant: pts with *PIK3CA* mutation, PFS 7.4 vs. 5.4 mo for fulvestrant alone (HR 0.70). SAE in 32% vs. 8.9% for fulvestrant alone (modest activity and toxicities do not support clinical use) (18).
			Buparlisib (pan-PI3K inhibitor)
			• BELLE-2, Phase 3, with fulvestrant: ITT-PFS 6.9 vs. 5 mo for placebo (HR 0.78), pts with *PIK3CA* mutation by ctDNA had greater treatment effect (PFS 7 vs. 3.2 mo for placebo; HR 0.76) (19)
			• BELLE-3, Phase 3, with fulvestrant and after mTOR inhibitor: ITT-PFS 3.9 vs. 1.8 mo for placebo (HR 0.67), pts with *PIK3CA* mutation had greater treatment effect (PFS 4.7 vs. 1.6 mo for placebo) (20)
			• BELLE-4, Phase 2, with paclitaxel. Median PFS 8.0 vs. 9.2 mo (ITT), Median PFS 9.1 vs. 9.2 mo (PI3K pathway activated). No treatment effect in ITT or pts with *PIK3CA* mutation (21).

(continued)

Actionable Target	Abnormality	Prevalence (%)	Clinical Experience with Targeted Agent
			Pictilisib (pan-PI3K inhibitor)
			• FERGI, Phase 2, with fulvestrant: no treatment effect in WT or *PIK3CA* mutation (22)
			• PEGGY, Phase 2, with paclitaxel: no treatment effect irrespective of *PIK3CA* mutation (23)
			Ipatasertib (selective Akt inhibitor)
			• Phase 1b, with paclitaxel: treatment effect in HER2− breast cancer including pts with PI3K/Akt alterations (24)
			• IPATUNITY 130 Cohort B, Phase 3, with paclitaxel: pts with PI3K/Akt1/PTEN alteration—no improvement in PFS (9.2 vs. 8.5 mo for placebo) (25)
			Capivasertib (selective Akt inhibitor)
			• BEECH, Phase 1/2, with paclitaxel: no improvement in PFS in overall population (10.9 vs. 8.4 mo for placebo) or in pts with *PIK3CA* mutation (10.9 vs. 10.8 mo for placebo) (26)
			• FAKTION, Phase 2, with fulvestrant: overall population with treatment effect—PFS 10.3 vs. 4.8 mo for placebo (HR 0.58), PI3K/PTEN alteration did not predict response—9.5 vs. 5.2 mo for placebo (27)

Actionable Target	Abnormality	Prevalence (%)	Clinical Experience with Targeted Agent
		HER2+: ~25%–30%	**HER2+** <ul><li>*PIK3CA* mutation associated with resistance to **trastuzumab** and shorter survival (28,29)</li><li>CLEOPATRA, Phase 3: Treatment effect to **pertuzumab** present in both WT and *PIK3CA* mutation; WT with greater treatment effect (PFS 21.8 WT vs. 12.5 mo for *PIK3CA* mutation) (30)</li><li>EMILIA, Phase 3: No difference in treatment effect with **T-DM1** based on WT or mutated *PIK3CA* (31)</li></ul> **Everolimus** (mTOR inhibitor) <ul><li>BOLERO-1, Phase 3, with trastuzumab and paclitaxel: ITT—no difference in PFS vs. placebo, pts with *PIK3CA* mutations and/or PTEN loss and/or Akt1 mutation with treatment effect—PFS 13.9 vs. 10.9 mo for placebo (HR 0.72) (32,33)</li><li>BOLERO-3, Phase 3, with trastuzumab and vinorelbine: ITT-PFS 7 vs. 5.8 mo for placebo (HR 0.78), pts with *PIK3CA* mutations and/or PTEN loss and/or Akt1 mutation with treatment effect—PFS 8.1 vs. 5.6 mo for placebo (HR 0.62) (33,34)</li><li>Some early-phase studies support PI3K inhibitor in combination with anti-HER2 therapy (35–38), but another study does not support efficacy (39)</li></ul> *(continued)*

Actionable Target	Abnormality	Prevalence (%)	Clinical Experience with Targeted Agent

		Triple negative: ~7%–10%	**Triple negative**
			• Higher prevalence in metaplastic breast cancer (~40%) (40,41) and luminal androgen receptor subtype (42)
			  o Phase 1, liposomal doxorubicin, bevacizumab, and temsirolimus or everolimus in metaplastic TNBC: improved ORR in pts with PIK3 pathway alteration (31% vs. 0% WT) (43)
			• *PIK3CA* mutation prevalent in luminal androgen receptor–positive molecular subtype (~40%) (42)
			Ipatasertib (selective Akt inhibitor)
			  o LOTUS, Phase 2, with paclitaxel: overall population—PFS 6.2 vs. 4.9 mo for placebo (HR 0.60), pts with *PIK3CA*/Akt1/PTEN alteration had greater treatment effect—PFS 9 vs. 4.9 mo for placebo (HR 0.44) (44)
			  o IPATUNITY 130 Cohort A, Phase 3, with paclitaxel: pts with PI3K/Akt1/PTEN alteration—no improvement in PFS (5.5 vs. 5.4 mo for placebo) (45)
			Capivasertib (selective Akt inhibitor)
			• PAKT, Phase 2, with paclitaxel: overall population—PFS 5.9 vs. 4.2 mo for placebo (HR 0.74), pts with *PIK3CA*/Akt1/PTEN alteration had greater treatment effect—PFS 9.3 vs. 3.7 mo for placebo (HR 0.30) (46)

CHAPTER 5

HER2 (ERBB2) Mutations

Niamh Coleman and Sarina A. Piha-Paul

HER2 (ERBB2) Mutations

Key points

- In addition to amplifications, activating mutations in *ERBB2* (*HER2*) have also been described in breast cancers (1). Typically, these mutations tend to occur in the absence of HER2 gene amplifications (2).

- Feedback between *HER2* and ER signaling has been hypothesized to be reciprocal, such that inhibition of either pathway may lead to upregulation and activation of the other pathway (3,4)

- Mutations in *HER2* lead to hyperactivation of the receptor via increased homo- or heterodimerization and activation of downstream signaling cascades, such as the PI3K and MAPK pathways, which promote oncogenesis (5)

- Somatic mutations in *HER2* occur in approximately 3% of breast cancers, predominantly in hormone receptor–positive (HR+) HER2− (HER2 non-amplified) subtype (6,7)

- *HER2* mutations are enriched in patients with prior endocrine therapy and in lobular histology, where the rate may be as high as 10% (8,9)

- *HER2* mutations can be observed in the extracellular, juxta/transmembrane, and kinase domains. Unlike other oncogenes (e.g., *BRAF* or *KRAS*) no single variant predominates and the distribution of mutations varies by tumor type (10).

- Location of the mutation is important: kinase domain mutations (e.g., Y772-A775dup) could predict for response to TKIs (such as neratinib), while extracellular domain mutations could predict for response/resistance to trastuzumab/pertuzumab (e.g., ERBB2 S310F mutation) (11,12)

- *HER2* mutations are also reported across other tumors including bladder cancer (13%), colorectal cancer (3%), and non–small cell lung cancer (3%) (13)
- *HER2* mutations have been implicated in resistance to endocrine therapy as well as HER2-directed therapy and are associated with worse prognosis (14–16)
- Preexisting concurrent activating *HER2* or *HER3* alterations have been associated with poor treatment outcome. Similarly, multiple activating *HER2* or *HER3* as well as gatekeeper alterations were observed at disease progression in patients who derived benefit from neratinib (17).
- Neratinib, an irreversible pan-HER kinase inhibitor, has been shown to overcome endocrine resistance in *HER2*-mutant breast cancer cell lines and xenograft models (18)
- Bispecific antibodies, antibody–drug conjugates, and small molecule inhibitors (e.g., trastuzumab deruxtecan, neratinib, and tucatinib) are currently being investigated in clinical trials in *HER2*-mutant, non-amplified metastatic breast cancer
- Additionally, HER2 peptide vaccine and CAR-T cells are also being investigated in early-phase clinical trials

Actionable Target	Abnormality	Prevalence (%)	Clinical Experience with Targeted Agent
HER2 (*ERBB2*)	Mutation	**Approx. 3% (up to 10% in lobular and/or endocrine-treated/ resistant)**	• Single-arm Phase 2—neratinib single-agent CBR (defined as CR/PR/SD ≥ 24 wks) 31%, including one CR, one PR, and three SD ≥24 wks. Median PFS was 16 (90% CI 8–31) wks (19). • Phase 2 SUMMIT basket trial—neratinib single-agent ORR (at week 8) 32% (breast cohort, n = 25) (20). Responses observed in both ER+ (30%, 6/20) and ER− (40%, 2/5) tumors, and in extracellular and kinase domains, as well as insertions in the kinase domain. PFS 3.5 mo, CBR 40%. • Phase 2 SUMMIT basket trial—neratinib in combination with fulvestrant (HR+), ORR 30%, CBR 46.8% (including 4 CR, 10 PR), PFS 5.4 mo, DOR 9.2 mo (17) • Phase 2 SUMMIT basket trial—neratinib in combination with trastuzumab and fulvestrant, ORR 39%, (5 PR, 0 CR) (21) • Phase 2 PlasmaMATCH—neratinib and fulvestrant: ORR 25% (1 CR, 4 PR), CBR 45%, DOR 5.7 mo, PFS 5.4 mo (22). Agreement between ctDNA digital PCR and targeted sequencing was 96%–99%; sensitivity of digital PCR ctDNA testing for mutations identified in tissue sequencing was 93% overall and 98% with contemporaneous biopsies (22). • Phase 2 study (NCT03412383)—single-agent pyrotinib: ORR 40% and CBR 60% (23).

CHAPTER 6

Akt1 and PTEN

Niamh Coleman and Funda Meric-Bernstam

Key points

- The PI3K–Akt–mTOR signaling pathway is one of the most deregulated pathways in cancer and is associated with the development and maintenance of numerous solid tumors (1–3)

- In breast cancer, dysregulation of PI3K–Akt–mTOR pathway is a common event in many distinct subsets, including HR+ disease, HER2-amplified, and triple-negative tumors

- Akt is a key effector of the PI3K–Akt–mTOR signaling cascade, which controls a number of key cellular processes, such as metabolism, motility, growth, and proliferation and supports the survival, expansion, and dissemination of cancer cells (4)

- Akt belongs to the family of serine/threonine kinases consisting of three isoforms (Akt1, Akt2, and Akt3), regulated upstream by the activation of PI3K, following growth factor stimulation. The three Akt isoforms are encoded by different genes with high-sequence homology and display a conserved protein structure (5).

- Enhanced activation of all the isoforms can be implicated in tumor development and progression, although their functional spectrum shows variety: Akt1 has a suggested role in cell proliferation and survival, while Akt2 exercises its control over metabolism, regulates cytoskeleton dynamics; and Akt3 is more dominant in brain tissues, implicated in mediating cell growth processes along with Akt1 (6)

- PTEN (phosphatase and tensin homolog) functions as a negative regulator of the PI3K/Akt/PTEN pathway: it acts as a tumor suppressor gene via numerous mechanisms, one of which is antagonizing the PI3K/Akt/mTOR signaling pathway by dephosphorylating phosphatidylinositol (3,4,5)-trisphosphate (PIP3). PIP3 functions as a secondary messenger in the PI3K pathway that binds and activates proteins that have a pleckstrin homology domain, such as Akt1, and triggers their activation and localization to the plasma membrane, promoting cellular proliferation and survival (7). Consequently, loss of PTEN leads to pathway activation.

- PI3K/Akt pathway aberrations have been identified in almost 40% of all solid tumors: PTEN loss by IHC occurs most frequently (30%), followed by mutations in *PIK3CA* (13%), PTEN (6%), and Akt (1%) (8)

- In breast cancers, mutations in *PIK3CA* are common events, occurring in 9% to 45% of breast cancer (Luminal A [45%], Luminal B [29%], HER2 enriched [39%], Basal 9%). PTEN loss of function occurs in 13% to 35% and *Akt* mutations (2%–4%) or *Akt* amplification (5%–10%) are also described (9). Five to 10% of ER+ MBC harbor somatic *PTEN* mutations (10).

- In an estimated 7% of ER+ breast cancers, pathway activation can occur through mutation in Akt1, predominantly Akt1^{E17K} ($\sim$80%). Here, signaling is constitutively activated through pathologic localization of Akt1 to the plasma membrane (11).

- The PI3K/Akt signaling pathway is frequently hyperactivated in TNBC due to *PIK3CA* or *Akt1* gain-of-function mutations and/or PTEN inactivation. Combined activating mutations in *PIK3CA* and *Akt1*, with inactivating *PTEN* mutations, occur in $\sim$25% to 30% of advanced TNBC (12,13).

- Germline PTEN loss-of-function mutations can lead to dominant Akt activation as a driving oncogenic event, for example, in Cowden-related breast tumors. Exceptional durable responses to Akt inhibition have been demonstrated in patients with breast cancer and germline PTEN mutations (14).

- Akt inhibitors can be classified into two classes based on their mode of inhibition, either ATP-competitive or allosteric inhibitors. ATP-competitive agents (e.g., capivasertib and ipatasertib) target the catalytic site of the active kinase in the PH-out conformation and prevent substrate phosphorylation, while allosteric inhibitors (e.g., ARQ092, miransertib, MK-2206) target an allosteric pocket within the PH domain/kinase domain interface that stabilizes the PH-in conformation (15).

- Significant responses were initially reported using capivasertib in patients with heavily pretreated Akt1 E17K mutant solid tumors in a basket study, which included 20 patients with ER+ metastatic breast cancer, where the objective response rate (ORR) was 20% and median PFS was 5.5 mo (16)

- The results of a subprotocol of NCI-Match trial confirmed the clinical activity of capivasertib in Akt1 E17K-mutated tumors as clinically significant ORR was achieved (ORR 28.6%), median PFS was 5.5 mo (17). Of patients with confirmed PR, seven had HR+/ERBB2− breast cancer, one had uterine leiomyosarcoma, and one had oncocytic parotid gland carcinoma. The majority of patients treated had either breast cancer (51%) or gynecologic cancers (31%).

- Capivasertib plus fulvestrant has also shown antitumor activity in heavily pretreated patients with PTEN-mutated ER+ metastatic breast cancer, particularly in patients with prior progression on fulvestrant (18). In this study, capivasertib was deemed tolerable and clinically active: the 24-wk clinical benefit rate was 42% and ORR was 21% in the 19 fulvestrant-pretreated patients.

- Ipatasertib is another potent and selective ATP-competitive pan-Akt kinase inhibitor where impressive durable response in combination with fulvestrant has been reported in heavily pretreated patients with Akt*1 E17K* mutant metastatic breast cancer (19,20)

- Akt inhibitors in development include TAS0612, a novel multikinase inhibitor of Akt, p70S6K, and p90RSK (21), and TAS-117, a highly potent and selective oral allosteric pan-Akt inhibitor, which has demonstrated some clinical efficacy in patients with breast cancer harboring *PIK3CA* H1047R and A1E17K mutations (22). Multiple trials are ongoing, including Phase 3 trials and studies exploring innovative Akt combinations.

Actionable Target	Abnormality	Prevalence (%)	Clinical Experience with Targeted Agent
Akt1	Mutation	Approx. 7% HR+ BC predominantly *Akt1E17K* (~80%)	**Akt Inhibitors in HR+/HER2− BC** • **Capivasertib:** in combination with fulvestrant Phase 1 in Akt1 E17K-mutant HR+ MBC; ORR in both fulvestrant-naïve (n = 15) and fulvestrant-pretreated (n = 28) pts, 20% and 36%, respectively (23). ≥50% decrease in Akt1^{E17K} at cycle 2 day 1 was associated with improved PFS. • **Capivasertib:** in combination with fulvestrant in randomized, placebo-controlled Phase 2 trial (FAKTION) in postmenopausal women with HR+/HER2− advanced BC postprogression AI: statistically significant 5.5 mo gain in median PFS (10.3 mo in the experimental arm vs. 4.8 mo in the control arm [HR 0.58; 95% CI 0.39–0.84, $p = 0.004$]) (24) • **Capivasertib:** in combination with weekly paclitaxel, Phase 1b/2 (BEECH): did not prolong PFS in the overall population or *PIK3CA+* subpopulation—median PFS 10.9 mo in experimental arm [n = 54] vs. 8.4 mo in the control arm [n = 56] [HR 0.80; $p = 0.308$]). In the *PIK3CA+* subpopulation, median PFS was 10.9 mo with capivasertib vs. 10.8 mo with placebo with paclitaxel (HR 1.11; $p = 0.760$) (25). *(continued)*

Actionable Target	Abnormality	Prevalence (%)	Clinical Experience with Targeted Agent
			• **TAS117:** single-agent preliminary data from Phase 2 (K-BASKET), 13 patients with advanced solid tumors harboring PI3K/Akt (12 patients showed mutations in PIK3 catalytic subunit alpha) (*PIK3CA*), 1 patient Akt1^{E17K}; 4 (31%) patients had breast cancer; 2 patients with breast cancer had stable disease, DCR of 23% (22) **Akt Inhibitors in TNBC** • **Capivasertib:** in combination with paclitaxel, randomized placebo-controlled Phase 2 trial (PAKT): ○ PFS was significantly extended in the *PIK3CA/*Akt1/PTEN-mutated subpopulation (9.3 vs. 3.7 mo; HR 0.3; 95% CI 0.11–0.79; $p = 0.1$). Favorable OS trend for capivasertib plus paclitaxel, regardless of mutational status, median OS 19.1 vs. 12.6 mo; HR 0.61; 95% CI 0.37–0.99; $p = 0.04$. Median OS NR vs. 10.4 mo: HR 0.37; 95% CI 0.12–1.12; $p = 0.07$, in PI3K altered subgroup (26). • Phase 3 randomized, placebo-controlled trial of capivasertib and paclitaxel for the first-line treatment of advanced TNBC (CAPItello290) opened for accrual in May 2020 (27)

Actionable Target	Abnormality	Prevalence (%)	Clinical Experience with Targeted Agent
			• **Ipatasertib:** in combination with paclitaxel, randomized placebo-controlled Phase 2 trial (LOTUS), PFS was significantly extended, PFS 6.2 vs. 4.9 mo; HR 0.6; 95% CI 0.37–0.98; $p = 0.03$; increase also in PTEN-low population (6.2 vs. 3.7 mo; HR 0.59; 95% CI 0.26–1.32; $p = 0.18$); ipatasertib benefit was more pronounced in the *PIK3CA*/Akt/PTEN-altered population ($n = 42$): median PFS was 9.0 vs. 4.9 mo in the control arm (HR 0·44; 95% CI 0.20–0.99, $p = 0.04$) (28) Update showed median OS was numerically longer with ipatasertib–paclitaxel than placebo–paclitaxel (HR 0.80, 95% CI 0.50–1.28; median 25.8 vs. 16.9 mo, respectively; 1-yr OS 83% vs. 68%), median OS favored ipatasertib–paclitaxel in the PTEN-low population (29)

(*continued*)

Actionable Target	Abnormality	Prevalence (%)	Clinical Experience with Targeted Agent
			• **Ipatasertib:** in combination with paclitaxel Phase 3 trial (IPATunity130 Cohort A) in pts with *PIK3CA*/Akt1/PTEN-altered TNBC did not significantly improve PFS (PFS 7.4 months [range, 5.6-8.5] in combination arm versus 6.1 months [range, 5.5-9.0] in the control arm [stratified HR 1.02; 95% CI, 0.71-1.45; log-rank $P = 0.9237$]). OS follow-up is ongoing. Safety was consistent with previously reported results. Results from this trial differ from findings in both randomized Phase 2 trials of Akt inhibition in TNBC (LOTUS and PAKT) (30) • **Ipatasertib:** in combination with a non-tax-ane–based chemotherapy in mTNBC patients is currently under evaluation in the Phase 2 PATHFINDER trial

Actionable Target	Abnormality	Prevalence (%)	Clinical Experience with Targeted Agent
PTEN	Mutation/loss	**5%–10%** ER+ BC **Approx. 50%** TNBC	5%–10% of ER+ metastatic breast cancer tumors harbor somatic PTEN mutations and loss of function of PTEN defines an aggressive, treatment-refractory subtype (31) • **Capivasertib:** in combination with fulvestrant Phase 1 multipart expansion study in pts with PTEN-mutant ER+ MBC, 24-wk CBR was 17% in fulvestrant naive (n = 12) and 42% in fulvestrant pretreated (n = 19); ORR of 8% and 21%, respectively (18) • **Ipatasertib** in combination with paclitaxel, Phase 2 (described above) with PFS 6.2 vs. 3.6 mo (paclitaxel), ORR 48% vs. 26% for PTEN low (28) • **Alpelisib** (alpha-selective PI3K inhibitor) in combination with fulvestrant, post hoc analyses of Phase 3 (SOLAR-1); in the small group of pts (n = 19) whose tumors had PTEN loss but no *PIK3CA* alteration, ALP showed an improved mPFS and favorable HR vs. the placebo arm: PFS 6.2 vs. 1.9 mo for fulvestrant alone in PTEN loss (without *PIK3CA* mutation), PFS 7.7 vs. 3.6 mo in PTEN loss (with *PIK3CA* mutation) (32)

CHAPTER 7

FGFR

Blessie Elizabeth Nelson and Jordi Rodon-Ahnert

Key points

- Fibroblast growth factor receptors (FGFRs) belong to the receptor tyrosine kinases (RTKs) family and play essential roles in mediating cell proliferation, migration, and survival (1)

- FGFR family includes four highly conserved RTKs—namely, *FGFR1*, *FGFR2*, *FGFR3*, and *FGFR4*— that are encoded by distinct genes, and an additional receptor named *FGFR5* (also known as *FGFRL1*), which lacks the intracellular kinase domain. The latter acts as a decoy receptor (2).

- The FGF ligands comprises a family of 22 conserved ligands, FGFs 1–10 and the FGFs 16–23, that act in paracrine or endocrine manner depending on the subtype (2)

- Deregulation of FGFR signaling pathway has been recognized in multiple cancers including breast, prostate, endometrial, and lung cancers (3)

- Aberrant FGFR signaling in cancers is mediated through *FGFR* amplifications, mutations, or rearrangements (3). Across tumors, *FGFR* amplifications are the most common (66%) followed by mutations (26%) and rearrangements (8%) (3).

- Amplifications in *FGFR1* and *FGFR2* are mainly observed in breast cancers, although rarely mutations and rearrangements in *FGFR* have also been reported (3–5)

- *FGFR1* amplification is observed in ~15% of breast cancers primarily in ER+ tumors. *FGFR2* is observed in <1% of breast but common in TNBC (~4%) (2).

- Coamplification of 8p11 and 11q13 with amplification of *CCND1*, *MYC* is typically observed in ER+ breast cancers (3,6)

- Alterations in FGFR pathway have been implicated in resistance to endocrine therapy and CDK4/6 inhibitors in breast cancers (7–10)

- Erdafitinib is approved in advanced urothelial carcinoma with *FGFR2/3* alterations, while pemigatinib and infigratinib have been approved in advanced cholangiocarcinoma with *FGFR2* fusion or rearrangements (11–13)

- Approximately 25% of cases with *FGFR1* amplifications also harbor *PIK3CA* alterations (3)

- PI3K/Akt/mTOR signaling pathway has been implicated in resistance to FGFR targeting (14)

- Currently there is no approved therapy for *FGFR* alterations in breast cancer and initial trials with nonselective FGFR inhibitors have yielded mixed results, although clinical trials are ongoing (15)

Actionable Target	Abnormality	Prevalence (%)	Clinical Experience with Targeted Agent
FGFR1	Amplification	10%–15%	• Predictive for response to FGFR inhibitors • **Phase 2:** Dovitinib monotherapy in MBC, unconfirmed PR, or SD ≥ 6 mo in 5/20 patients. ORR ~ 20% in patients with ≥6 copies of FGFR1 (16). • **Phase 2:** Dovitinib in combination with fulvestrant vs. fulvestrant in MBC. PFS 10.9 vs. 5.5 mo (HR 0.64) in FGF pathway-amplified subgroup (17). • **Phase 1:** BGJ398 in solid tumors, no PR, SD in ~30% (18) • **Phase 2 MATCH Trial:** AZD4547 in tumors with FGFR alterations. PR 8% in tumors with FGFR1-3 mutations or fusions. No significant clinical benefit in patients with FGFR1-amplified breast cancer. • **Phase 1:** Debio 1347 in combination with fulvestrant in MBC. Disease stabilization in 1/7 patients with high FGFR1 amplification (19). • **Phase 2:** Lucitanib in MBC. ORR 19% in FGFR1 amplified. ORR 22% in high FGFR1 amplifications (≥4 copies) vs. 9% in low. ORR 25% in FGFR1-high (IHC, H-score ≥ 50) vs. 8% in FGFR1-low (20)

CHAPTER 8

NTRK

Senthil Damodaran and Debu Tripathy

Key points

- The tropomyosin-related kinases (TRKs) are neurotrophin receptors that belong to the tyrosine receptor kinase family and consist of three members: TRKA, TRKB, and TRKC, which are encoded by *NTRK1*, *NTRK2*, and *NTRK3*, respectively (1)

- TRK receptor family is involved in neuronal growth and differentiation. TRK receptors dimerize and phosphorylate each other in response to ligand, leading to downstream activation of MAPK, PI3K, and PLCγ pathways.

- Recurrent chromosomal fusion events involving the carboxy-terminal kinase domain of TRK, and various upstream amino-terminal partners have been reported across diverse cancers in children and adults such as congenital fibrosarcoma, papillary thyroid, colon, and lung cancer

- While rare in breast cancers, activating *NTRK* fusions are primarily observed in secretory breast cancers, a rare, triple-negative subtype which is characterized by a pathognomonic *ETV6-NTRK3* fusion (2). *NTRK* fusions have also been reported in other subtypes including lobular and metaplastic tumors (3).

- While *ETV6* appears to be the primary partner for *NTRK3*, *NTRK1* appears to involve a variety of fusion partners including *MDM4*, *LMNA*, *PEAR1*, and *TMP3* (3,4)

- In addition to *NTRK* rearrangements, *NTRK* amplifications and *NTRK* mutations have also been described. However, the actionability of these non-fusion *NTRK* alterations is not well established with study showing limited benefit in such patients (5). *NTRK* mutations have been shown to mediate acquired resistance to entrectinib in patients harboring *NTRK* fusions (6).

- Clinical trial evaluating the activity of larotrectinib in patients with *NTRK* amplifications is ongoing (NCT04879121)

Actionable Target	Abnormality	Prevalence (%)	Clinical Experience with Targeted Agent
NTRK	Fusion	<1	**Entrectinib** • 83% ORR breast cancers (7) • Tumor agnostic FDA approval for tumor types with *NTRK* fusions **Larotrectinib** • Tumor agnostic FDA approval for tumor types with *NTRK* fusions (8) • 83% ORR in breast cancers. 100% ORR in TNBC with *NTRK3* or *NTRK1* fusion (4).

CHAPTER 9

HER2 Amplifications

Senthil Damodaran and Debu Tripathy

HER2 Amplifications

Key points

- *ERRB2* is amplified and overexpressed in 15% to 20% of breast cancers. HER2 belongs to the ERBB protein kinase superfamily, which also includes epidermal growth factor receptor (EGFR [ERBB1]), HER3 (ERBB3), and HER4 (ERBB4) (1).

- HER2 overexpression results in augmented signaling through downstream PI3K and MAPK pathways leading to activation of proto-oncogenes and transcriptional factors such as fos, jun, myc, and increased cell survival and proliferation (1)

- Unlike other ERBB family members that require ligand binding for activation, signaling through HER2 occurs in the absence of a known ligand, while dimerization with self and other ERBB family member modulates downstream signaling

- HER2 overexpression has been shown to confer intrinsic resistance to endocrine therapy, signifying the interaction between hormone receptors and the EGFR family (2,3)

- HER2 amplification/overexpression is observed in nearly half of all in situ ductal carcinomas, particularly in high-grade tumors (4). However, use of trastuzumab concurrently with radiation did not achieve a significant reduction in ipsilateral breast tumor recurrence (IBTR) (5).

- Multiple HER2 targeting agents have been approved for clinical use
  - Trastuzumab is a recombinant humanized monoclonal antibody (mAb) that binds with high affinity to the extracellular juxta membrane domain IV of HER2
  - Pertuzumab is the recombinant mAb that binds to the dimerization arm (extracellular domain II) of HER2, resulting in the disruption of HER2:HER3 heterodimer
  - Trastuzumab emtansine (T-DM1) is an antibody–drug conjugate (ADC) with trastuzumab linked to the cytotoxic microtubule inhibitor DM-1

- Trastuzumab deruxtecan (T-DXd) is ADC composed of a humanized anti-HER2 IgG1 mAb (MAAL-9001) with the same amino acid sequence as trastuzumab, covalently linked to a topoisomerase inhibitor (MAAA-1181a, DXd) via a tetrapeptide-based cleavable linker. T-DXd has a higher drug-to-antibody ratio than T-DM1 (~8 vs. 3–4).
  - Lapatinib is an oral, reversible TKI that targets the ATP binding site located on the intracellular kinase domains of both EGFR and HER2
  - Neratinib is an irreversible TKI that binds to EGFR, HER2, and HER4
  - Tucatinib is an oral, highly selective inhibitor of HER2
  - Margetuximab-cmkb is a chimeric, Fc-engineered, IgG1 HER2 mAb that shares epitope specificity and Fc-independent antiproliferative effects with trastuzumab with increased affinity for activating Fcγ receptor CD16A (FcγRIIIa) and decreased affinity for inhibitory FcγR CD32B (FcγRIIIb)

- Activating mutations in HER2 have been reported in MBC and are typically exclusive with HER2 amplifications, and are more common in hormone receptor–positive cases and after prolonged exposure to endocrine therapy (6)

- Activation of PI3K pathway (e.g., *PIK3CA* mutations or PTEN loss) has been shown to be associated with resistance to HER2-directed therapies (7,8)

Actionable Target	Abnormality	Prevalence (%)	Clinical Experience with Targeted Agent
ERBB2 (*HER2*)	Amplification	20%	**Trastuzumab** (HER2 inhibitor) (FDA approved): • Phase 3: Single agent, first line, ORR 26% (9) • Phase 3, with **chemotherapy (**anthracycline based or paclitaxel): ORR 50% vs. 32% for chemo alone, PFS 7.4 vs. 4.6 mo (10) • Phase 2, APT trial, with weekly paclitaxel, for tumors <3 cm, node negative, 7-yr disease-free survival 93%, relapse-free interval 97.5% (11) • Phase 3, with **lapatinib**, neoadjuvant: ORR 51% vs. 30% with trastuzumab alone vs. 24% with lapatinib alone (12) **Lapatinib** (dual HER2/EGFR inhibitor) (FDA approved): • Phase 2: Single agent, after trastuzumab, ORR 7.7%, CBR 14.1 wks (13) • Phase 3, with **trastuzumab**: PFS 12 vs. 8.1 mo for lapatinib, HR = 0.73, $p = 0.008$, CBR 24.7% vs. 12.4%, OS 14 vs. 9.5 mo (14,15) • Phase 3, with **capecitabine**: PFS 8.4 vs. 4.1 mo for capecitabine, ORR 22 vs. 14 mo (16) **Pertuzumab** (HER2 dimerization inhibitor) (FDA approved): • Phase 3, CLEOPATRA study, with **trastuzumab** and **docetaxel**: PFS 18.5 vs. 12.4 mo with trastuzumab and docetaxel (HR 0.62, $p < 0.001$), ORR 80% vs. 69%, OS 56.5 vs. 40.8 mo (HR 0.68, $p < 0.001$) (17,18)

Actionable Target	Abnormality	Prevalence (%)	Clinical Experience with Targeted Agent
			• Single agent, ORR 3.4% (19). With **trastuzumab**, ORR 17.6% (19) • Phase 3, APHINITY with adjuvant trastuzumab: 3-yr IDFS 94.1% with pertuzumab vs. 93.2% with trastuzumab alone. In node-positive, 3-yr IFDS 92% vs. 90.2% (HR 0.77, $p = 0.02$). 6-yr IDFS in node-positive, 88% vs. 83%. No benefit in node negative (20,21). **T-DM1 (ado-trastuzumab emtansine)** (antibody–drug conjugate to HER2; trastuzumab linked with emtansine) (FDA approved): • Phase 3: EMILIA, PFS 9.6 vs. 6.4 mo (HR 0.65, $p < 0.001$) for lapatinib and capecitabine. OS 30.9 vs. 25.1 mo (HR 0.68, $p < 0.001$). ORR 44% vs. 31% (22). • Phase 3: TH3RESA, PFS 6.2 vs. 3.3 mo for treatment of physician's choice (HR 0.528, $p < 0.0001$), third line or greater (23) **Neratinib** (Pan ERRB2 inhibitor) (FDA approved): • Phase 3, ExteNET study, after adjuvant trastuzumab: 2-yr IDFS 93.9% vs. 91.6% with placebo. 5-yr IDFS 90.2% vs. 87.7% (HR 0.73, $p = 0.0083$) (24,25).

(continued)

Actionable Target	Abnormality	Prevalence (%)	Clinical Experience with Targeted Agent
			• Phase 3, for metastatic BC (FDA approved): **With capecitabine**, Mean PFS 8.8 vs. 6.6 mo (lapatinib and capecitabine) (HR 0.76, $p = 0.0059$). OS 24 vs. 22.2 mo (HR 0.88, $p = 0.2086$), ORR 33% vs. 27% (26). **Trastuzumab deruxtecan (DS-8201)** (topoisomerase inhibitor drug conjugate to HER2) (FDA approved): • Phase 2: DESTINY-Breast01, ORR 61%, CR 6%, DOR 14.8 mo (27) • Phase 3: DESTINY-Breast03, median PFS 25.1 vs. 7.2 mo for T-DM1, ORR 79.1% vs. 34.2%. Median treatment duration 14.3 vs. 6.9 mo (28). **Tucatinib** (selective HER2 inhibitor) (FDA approved): • Phase 2: in combination with trastuzumab and capecitabine, PFS 7.8 vs. 5.6 mo (trastuzumab and capecitabine alone), OS 21.9 vs. 17.4 mo, ORR 41% vs. 23% (29). Median CNS-PFS 9.9 vs. 4.2 mo (30).

Actionable Target	Abnormality	Prevalence (%)	Clinical Experience with Targeted Agent
			Margetuximab (Fc-modified trastuzumab analog) (FDA approved) • Phase 3: Compared trastuzumab vs. margetuximab with chemotherapy of choice (capecitabine, eribulin, gemcitabine, or vinorelbine), PFS 5.8 vs. 4.9 mo (HR = 0.76, $p = 0.03$), ORR 25% vs. 14% (trastuzumab with chemotherapy) (31) **SYD985** (ADC based on trastuzumab and a cleavable linker-duocarmicin [vc-*seco*-DUBA] payload) • Phase 3: SYD985 vs. treatment of physician's choice (trastuzumab with capecitabine, trastuzumab with capecitabine, trastuzumab with vinorelbine, trastuzumab with eribulin, or lapatinib with capecitabine), PFS 6.9 vs. 4.6 mo (HR 0.60, $p < 0.001$), OS 20.4 vs. 16.3 mo (HR 0.83, $p = 0.153$)

CHAPTER 10

PD-1/PD-L1/MSI/TMB

Haven Garber

Key points

- The immune checkpoint receptor PD-1 and its major ligand PD-L1 are primary targets of cancer immunotherapy. Their therapeutic blockade has demonstrated anticancer activity across tumor types (1).

- Checkpoint inhibitors, in combination with chemotherapy, have mediated incremental improvements in response rates and in progression-free and overall survival in a subset of patients with TNBC (2–4)

- Response rates in patients with hormone receptor–positive, HER2− disease have been disappointing (5,6)

- The relative potency of checkpoint inhibitors in patients with TNBC (vs. other breast cancer subtypes) correlates with higher tumor-infiltrating lymphocytes (TILs) and higher PD-L1 expression (7–11)

- Atezolizumab received accelerated approval from the FDA in 2019 for patients with metastatic PD-L1+ TNBC based on the IMpassion130 trial (3); however, the company voluntarily withdrew TNBC as an indication for the drug in August 2021 (12)

- As of November 2021, pembrolizumab is the only checkpoint inhibitor with FDA approval for patients with TNBC. There are no checkpoint inhibitors approved for hormone receptor–positive or HER2+ breast cancer. Pembrolizumab is indicated for patients with stage II/III TNBC in combination with neoadjuvant chemotherapy, regardless of PD-L1 status (13). It is also indicated in combination with chemotherapy for patients with metastatic PD-L1+ TNBC (CPS $\geq$ 10, 22C3 Ab) (2).

- There are numerous ongoing clinical trials across breast cancer subtypes that aim to build on the success of PD-1/PD-L1 checkpoint inhibitors by combining them with agents targeting additional immune checkpoints or signaling pathways including LAG3, OX40, 4-1BB, the VEGF pathway, and DNA damage response pathways (14–16)

Actionable Target	Abnormality	Prevalence (%)	Clinical Experience with Targeted Agent
PD-1/PD-L1	Overexpression	~40% of tumors in patients with metastatic TNBC are PD-L1+: CPS ≥10 (22C3 Ab)[a] or PD-L1 ≥1% (SP142 Ab)[b]	**Pembrolizumab** (PD-1 inhibitor): • Phase 3 (metastatic): Frontline pembro + chemo vs. chemo alone; 22C3 Ab; in **CPS ≥10**, **PFS** 9.7 vs. 5.6 mo (HR 0.65, 95% CI 0.49–0.86, $p = 0.0014$), ORR 53.2% vs. 39.8%; in CPS ≥1, **PFS** 7.6 vs. 5.6 mo (HR 0.74, 95% CI 0.61–0.9, ns), ORR 45.2% vs. 37.9%; in ITT, **PFS** 7.5 vs. 5.6 mo (HR 0.82, 95% CI 0.69–0.97, not tested), ORR 41% vs. 35.9%; median OS (CPS ≥ 10) 23 vs. 16.1 mo (HR 0.73 [0.55–0.95] $p = 0.0093$), met prespecified boundary of 0.0113 (17). This trial (KEYNOTE-355) led to FDA approval of pembro in PD-L1+ (CPS ≥ 10) mTNBC (2) • Phase 3 (neoadjuvant): neoadj pembro + chemo (and adj pembro) vs. neoadj chemo alone; **pCR** 64.8% vs. 51.2%, $p = 0.00055$; in ITT, 3-yr **EFS** 84.5% vs. 76.8%, HR 0.63 (95% CI 0.48–0.82, $p = 0.00031$); if yes pCR, 3-yr EFS 94.4% vs. 92.5%, if no pCR, 3-yr EFS 67.4% vs. 56.8%; EFS benefit seen in PD-L1+ and PD-L1 tumors; OS data immature, this trial (KEYNOTE-522) led to FDA approval of pembro in early-stage TNBC regardless of PD-L1 status (13,18) *(continued)*

Actionable Target	Abnormality	Prevalence (%)	Clinical Experience with Targeted Agent
			• Phase 2 (metastatic): PD-L1+ patients (CPS ≥ 1), pembro as frontline treatment, ORR 21.4% (19) • Phase 3 (metastatic): pembro vs. chemo as 2nd or 3rd line treatment for TNBC, no sig difference in OS (20) **Atezolizumab** (PD-L1 inhibitor): • Phase 3 (metastatic): Frontline atezo + nab-paclitaxel vs. nab-paclitaxel alone; in ITT, **PFS** 7.2 vs. 5.5 mo (HR 0.8, 95% CI 0.69–0.92, $p = 0.002$), ORR 56% vs. 45.9%; in PD-L1+ (SP142, ≥1%), **PFS** 7.5 vs. 5 mo (HR 0.62, 95% CI 0.49–0.78, $p < 0.001$), ORR 58.9% vs. 42.6%; in ITT, **OS** 21 vs. 18.7 mo (HR 0.87, 95% CI 0.75–1.02, ns); in PD-L1+ **OS** 25.4 vs. 17.9 mo (HR 0.67, 95% CI 0.53–0.86, not formally tested due to hierarchical design), this study (IMpassion130) led to FDA approval of atezo for PD-L1+ mTNBC; however, the approval was later withdrawn (4,12,21)

Actionable Target	Abnormality	Prevalence (%)	Clinical Experience with Targeted Agent
			• Phase 3 (metastatic): Frontline atezo + paclitaxel vs. paclitaxel alone; in PD-L1+ (SP142), **PFS** 6 vs. 5.7 mo (HR 0.82, 95% CI 0.6–1.12, ns), failure to meet this post-marketing FDA requirement contributed to the withdrawal of atezo for mTNBC (12) • Phase 3 (neoadjuvant): Atezo + neoadj chemo vs. chemo alone; pCR 58% vs. 41% (EFS data immature) (22) **Durvalumab** (PD-L1 inhibitor): • Phase 2 (neoadjuvant): durva + neoadj chemo vs. chemo alone; pCR 53.4% vs. 44.2%; 3 yr iDFS 84.9% vs. 76.9% (23) **Avelumab** (PD-L1 inhibitor): • Phase 1 (metastatic, prior treatment): ORR 5.2% PR in TNBC (6)

(*continued*)

Actionable Target	Abnormality	Prevalence (%)	Clinical Experience with Targeted Agent
MSI-high/ dMMR or TMB-H (≥10 mutations/ Mb)		~1%–2% of all breast cancers (similar prevalence for TNBC)	**Pembrolizumab** • FDA approved for MSI-H or dMMR cancers (24,25); 2 of the 149 patients in the registration studies had breast cancer • FDA approved for tumor mutational burden-high (TMB-H) ≥10 mutations/Mb, no patients with breast cancer were included in the registration study (KEYNOTE-158) (26–29) • Phase 2: metastatic breast cancer patients with TMB-H, ORR 21%, median PFS 10.6 wks (30)

[a]The PD-L1 22C3 immunohistochemistry assay was used in KEYNOTE-355 (2) and KEYNOTE-522 (13) to assess the activity of pembrolizumab in patient subgroups.

[b]The PD-L1 SP142 immunohistochemistry assay was used in IMpassion130 (3) and IMpassion131 (31) to assess the activity of atezolizumab in patient subgroups. FDA accelerated approval for atezolizumab has since been withdrawn for metastatic TNBC (12). The PD-L1 assays are not interchangeable (32).

CHAPTER 11

TROP-2

Senthil Damodaran and Funda Meric-Bernstam

TROP-2

Key points

- TROP-2 (trophoblast cell-surface antigen 2) is a 36-kDa transmembrane glycoprotein and calcium signal transducer encoded by *TACSTD2* (Tumor-Associated Calcium Signal Transducer 2) (1)

- Trop-2 plays a major role in cell proliferation, survival, and invasion (2)

- Trop-2 is overexpressed in multiple tumors including breast, lung, colon, gastric, and ovary and is associated with aggressive disease and poor prognosis (3–6)

- Sacituzumab govitecan is an anti-Trop-2 humanized IgG1κ mAb connected to SN-38, the active metabolite irinotecan, through a maleimide–polyethylene glycol–acid-sensitive cleavable (carbonate) linker (3)

- Sacituzumab govitecan is approved for unresectable locally advanced or metastatic TNBC who have received two or more prior systemic therapies, at least one of them for metastatic disease (7)

- While sacituzumab govitecan showed clinical activity in patients with metastatic TNBC, irrespective of Trop-2 expression, greater efficacy was observed in those who had a medium or high Trop-2 score (8)

- Uridine diphosphate glucuronosyltransferase 1A1 (UGT1A1) is involved in the metabolism of SN-38 to SN-glucuronide, consequently concomitant administration of drugs that alter UGT1A1 activity should be avoided to minimize the potential for severe adverse effects (7)

- Patients homozygous for the UGT1A1"28 allele are at an increased risk for adverse reactions, especially neutropenia (~20% of the Black or African American population, compared with 10% of the White population, are homozygous for the UGT1A1"28 allele) (7)
- Sacituzumab has also shown promising activity in HR+ MBC and confirmatory clinical studies are in progress (9,10)
- Datopotamab deruxtecan (data-dxd) is a humanized anti-TROP-2 IgG1 mAb attached to a topoisomerase I inhibitor payload, an exatecan derivative, via a tetrapeptide-based cleavable linker (11)
- Trials evaluating Trop-2 targeted agents with immunotherapy and other targeted therapy are currently in progress (12)

Actionable Target	Abnormality	Prevalence (%)	Clinical Experience with Targeted Agent
TROP-2	Overexpression	~90%	**Sacituzumab Govitecan (FDA approved)** • **Phase 3, ASCENT trial**, sacituzumab vs. chemotherapy of physician's choice (eribulin, vinorelbine, capecitabine, or gemcitabine). PFS 5.6 vs. 1.7 mo (HR 0.41, $p < 0.001$), OS 12.1 vs. 6.7 mo (HR 0.48, $p < 0.001$), ORR 35% vs. 5% (13). • Median PFS was 6.9, 5.6, and 2.7 mo in high, medium, and low Trop-2 expression respectively. Median OS was 14.2 mo in high, 14.9 mo in medium, and 9.3 mo low Trop-2 expression (8). • **Phase 1/2 trial in HR+ MBC** (prespecified analysis), with prior progression on endocrine therapy and one line of chemotherapy, ORR 31.5%, median PFS 5.5 mo, median OS 12 mo (9) **Datopotamab Deruxtecan** • Phase 1, TROPION-Pantumor01 study, TNBC cohort—ORR 34% in all comers and 52% in patients without prior exposure to Topo-1 inhibitor–based ADC therapies (11)

Molecular Diagnostics and Testing

Current advances in molecular techniques and bioinformatics have enabled the detection of actionable genetic alterations for breast cancers and other solid tumors. Genomic alteration provides prognostic and predictive information to guide standard and investigational targeted therapeutic regimens as well as to discern mechanisms of resistance to therapy. Matching therapies that target single-nucleotide variations (SNVs), gene fusions (translocations), or copy number variations (CNVs) have been Food and Drug Administration (FDA) approved across various tumor types. In sporadic cases, somatic mutations and other alterations can be detected in tumor tissue and/or circulating tumor DNA. In hereditary breast cancer patients, germline mutations are detected in normal tissue or peripheral blood. Multiple DNA- and RNA-based assays are currently available to detect the actionable genomic alterations in breast cancer. The molecular tests can be personalized according to the tumor histology, immunophenotype, and tumor stage to assist efficient identification of actionable alterations to guide targeted therapy.

MOLECULAR TESTING PLATFORMS

In situ hybridization (ISH) is used to determine a specific DNA or RNA sequence in a tissue section (in situ) using a labeled complementary DNA, RNA, or modified nucleic acid probe. It can be used to detect deletions, amplifications, and translocations/fusions. ISH techniques include chromogenic ISH, which uses brightfield microscopes for label detection, and fluorescence in situ hybridization (FISH), which uses fluorescence microscopes for label detection (Figure 2.1).

    Immunohistochemistry (IHC) utilizes antibodies to bind proteins to assess protein expression levels in tissues.

    Polymerase chain reaction (PCR) is used to amplify and detect DNA and RNA sequences. Standard PCR involves the amplification of one or more copies of a chosen DNA sequence to produce millions of copies and enable detection and analysis. Reverse transcription (RT)-PCR converts RNA templates into complementary DNA for molecular analysis.

Figure 2.1

67

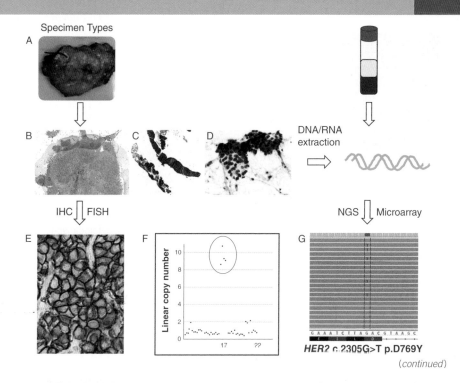

Specimen Types

A

B

C

D

DNA/RNA extraction

IHC | FISH

NGS | Microarray

E

F

G

Linear copy number

10

8

6

4

2

17   ??

G A A A T C T T A G A C G T A A G C

HER2 c.2305G>T p.D769Y

(continued)

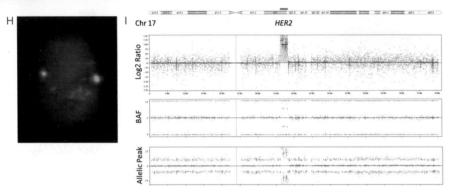

Breast cancer biomarker testing samples and assays. The testing samples include histologic specimens from surgical resection **(A and B)** and core needle biopsy **(C)**, cytologic specimens from fine-needle aspiration **(D)** and exfoliative specimen, and circulating free DNA from peripheral blood. Representative images illustrate HER2 testing by immunohistochemistry (IHC) for HER2 overexpression **(E)**, next-generation sequencing (NGS) for HER2 amplification **(F)**, NGS for HER2 mutation **(G)**, fluorescence in situ hybridization (FISH) for HER2 amplification **(H)**, and SNP array for HER2 amplification **(I)**.

The application of next-generation sequencing (NGS) to characterize cancer genomes has enabled the discovery of numerous predictive and prognostic breast cancer markers and the detection of actionable genetic alterations for breast cancer patients. The DNA-based NGS assays allow for the detection of single-nucleotide variant (SNV), short insertion, deletions (indels), and copy number alterations (CNAs), whereas RNA-based assays can detect fusion, splice variants, and RNA expression.

The available technologies enable the design of various NGS assays for different clinical settings (Table 2.1). The library of the targeted sequences can be generated by the hybrid capture chemistry or amplicon-based multiplex PCR. Massively parallel sequencing can be performed by different technologies, such as fluorescent reversible terminator–based sequencing-by-synthesis used in Illumina platforms, semiconductor-based sequencing used in Thermo Fisher platforms, and single-molecule real-time (SMRT) sequencing used in Pacific Biosciences platform. The hybrid capture chemistry is coupled with bridge amplification and fluorescent reversible terminator–based sequencing within the flow cells in the majority of Illumina assays. The fluorescent reversible terminator–based sequencing has a high confidence in sequencing accuracy for mutation detection. In the earlier designs, these assays required much higher DNA input than that required for the semiconductor-based sequencing assay used in Thermo Fisher platforms; therefore, the previous Illumina panels precluded extremely small samples to be sequenced. With the advances in assay design, the DNA input in the current Illumina panels has significantly decreased, allowing small biopsy samples to be tested. The semiconductor-based sequencing detects the nucleotide incorporation by measuring the change of pH because of proton released from the 3′-hydroxyl group during nucleotide incorporation; therefore, sequencing is rapid. However, the error rate is high in homopolymer regions if the sophisticated bioinformatic correction is not applied.

The choice of NGS assay is dependent on the coverage and the desired markers for selection of matching targeted therapies as standard or for clinical trial enrollment. Commercial NGS panels are built to accommodate targets across tumors, variants, and gene coverage (Table 2.1). Smaller panels tend to focus on hotspot somatic mutations of common oncogenes and tumor suppressors, for example, *ERBB2(HER2)*, *PIK3CA*, and *TP53*, in Ion AmpliSeq Cancer Hotspot Panel v2 (50-gene) and TruSeq Amplicon Cancer Panel (48-gene). The large-size panels contain pan-cancer biomarker

Table 2.1 Molecular Diagnostic Assays

Platforms and Assay Specification	Sample Type	Nucleic Acid	Input	Variant Class	Provider/Vendor
Next-Generation Sequencing by Reversible Terminator-Based Sequencing-by-Synthesis • High confidence					
TruSeq Amplicon Cancer Panel (48-gene) • Amplicon based • Amplicon size 170–190 bp • Limit of detection: 5% VAF	FFPE	DNA	250 ng	SNV, small indels	Illumina
TruSight Tumor 170 (170-gene) • Hybrid capture • Minimum insert size 79 bp for DNA and 63 bp for RNA • Limit of detection: 5% mutant allele frequency with ≥250× minimum coverage • Sensitivity and specificity >95%	FFPE	DNA, RNA	40 ng	SNV, indels, CNV, fusion, splice variant	Illumina
TruSight Oncology 500 (523-gene) • Hybrid capture • Limit of detection: 5% VAF • Analytical sensitivity >96% • Analytical specificity ≥9.9998%	FFPE	DNA, RNA	40 ng	SNV, indels, CNV, fusion, splice variant, MSI, TMB	Illumina

Table 2.1 Molecular Diagnostic Assays (*continued*)

71

Platforms and Assay Specification	Sample Type	Nucleic Acid	Input	Variant Class	Provider/ Vendor
TruSight Oncology 500 ctDNA (523-gene) • Mechanism of action: Hybrid capture chemistry • Limit of detection: 0.5% VAF • Analytical sensitivity and specificity ≥95%	Blood	cfDNA, ctDNA	30 ng	SNV, indels, CNV, fusion, splice variant, MSI, TMB	Illumina
Guardant360 CDx (73-gene) • Hybrid capture chemistry • Limit of detection: 0.3% VAF • Analytical sensitivity ≥95% • Analytical specificity ≥97%	Blood	cfDNA, ctDNA	10–30 ng	SNV, indels, CNV, fusion	Guardant Health
Next-Generation Sequencing by Semiconductor-Based Sequencing-by-Synthesis • Rapid sequencing rate • Limitation in homopolymer region					
Ion AmpliSeq Cancer Hotspot Panel v2 (50-gene) • Amplicon based • Amplicon size 111–187 bp • Limit of detection: 5% VAF	FFPE, cytology	DNA	10 ng	SNV	Thermo Fisher (*continuod*)

Table 2.1 Molecular Diagnostic Assays (*continued*)

Platforms and Assay Specification	Sample Type	Nucleic Acid	Input	Variant Class	Provider/ Vendor
Ion AmpliSeq Comprehensive Panel (409-gene) • Amplicon based • Amplicon size 125–175 bp • Limit of detection: 5% VAF	FFPE, cytology, blood	DNA	40 ng	SNV, indels, CNV	Thermo Fisher
Oncomine Comprehensive Assay v3 (161-gene) • Amplicon based • Amplicon size: median ~110 bp • Limit of detection: 5% VAF	FFPE, cytology	DNA, RNA	20 ng	SNV, indels, CNV, fusion, splice variant	Thermo Fisher
Next-Generation Sequencing by Anchored Multiplex PCR (AMP)					
FusionPlex Solid (53-gene)	FFPE	RNA	10 ng	Fusion, splice variant	Invitae
Single-Nucleotide Polymorphism Microarray					
OncoScan CNV Assay • Genome-wide structural variants such as deletions, duplications, LOH, cnLOH, break point determination, ploidy, mosaicism, and unbalanced translocations	FFPE, cytology	DNA	80 ng	CNV, LOH	Thermo Fisher

Table 2.1 Molecular Diagnostic Assays (*continued*)   73

Platforms and Assay Specification	Sample Type	Nucleic Acid	Input	Variant Class	Provider/ Vendor
RNA Expression Profile					
MammaPrint (70-gene) by RNA Microarray • Tumor <5 cm, 0–3 node positive • Prognostic for early distant recurrence in first 5 years • Predictive for chemo response in poor prognostic group	FFPE of primary tumor	RNA		RNA expression	Agendia
Oncotype DX (21-gene) by qRT-PCR • ER positive, 0–3 node positive • Recurrence score • Prognostic for distant recurrence in 10 years • Predictive for chemo response in high-recurrence score group	FFPE of primary tumor	RNA		RNA expression	Exact Sciences
Prosigna [PAM50] (50-gene) by qRT-PCR • Stages I–III • Prognostic based on assigned intrinsic molecular subtypes • Predictive for tamoxifen benefit in luminal cancers	FFPE of primary tumor	RNA		RNA expression	NanoString Technologies (*continued*)

Table 2.1 Molecular Diagnostic Assays (*continued*)

Platforms and Assay Specification	Sample Type	Nucleic Acid	Input	Variant Class	Provider/ Vendor
EndoPredict (12-gene) by qRT-PCR • ER positive, 0–3 node positive • Prognostic for late (5–10 years) distant recurrence after hormonal therapy	FFPE of primary tumor	RNA		RNA expression	Myriad Genetics Inc.
Germline Testing by Next-Generating Sequencing					
Myriad myRisk Hereditary Cancer (over 35-gene) • Detection of germline variants • Functional interpretation: deleterious mutation; genetic variant, suspected deleterious; genetic variant of uncertain significance; genetic variant, favor polymorphism; or genetic variant polymorphism	Blood, saliva	Germline DNA		SNV, indels, CNV	Myriad Genetics Inc.

cfDNA, circulating free DNA; cnLOH, copy-neutral LOH; CNV, copy number variation; ctDNA, circulating tumor DNA; ER, estrogen receptor; FFPE, formalin-fixed paraffin-embedded; LOH, loss of heterozygosity; MSI, microsatellite instability; qRT-PCR, quantitative reverse transcription polymerase chain reaction; SNV, single-nucleotide variant; TMB, tumor mutational burden; VAF, variant allele fraction.

content aligned with key clinical practice guidelines and clinical trials for solid tumor types, with both DNA and RNA assays targeting hundreds of genes for the assessment of variants for targeted therapy, and key immuno-oncology biomarkers such as microsatellite instability (MSI) status and tumor mutational burden (TMB). The comprehensive breast cancer–related genes such as *BRCA1*, *BRCA2*, and *MED2* are only included in intermediate- and large-size solid tumor panels such as Oncomine Comprehensive Assay v3 (161-gene), TruSight Tumor 170, and TruSight Oncology 500 panels. Panels with broad coverage potentially increase the chances of finding actionable biomarker(s) by moving from individual biomarker assays to a single comprehensive NGS assay.

Although high-throughput approaches such as whole-exome sequencing (WES) and transcriptome sequencing offer a more comprehensive genomic profile, because of limitations in cost and time, targeted gene panels are typically employed in clinical practice. Targeted panels employ select genes that are well characterized in terms of cancer biology and clinical relevance. In addition to cost advantage, targeted panels offer a faster turnaround time and scalability to meet standards for clinical grade testing such as Clinical Laboratory Improvement Amendments (CLIA) and College of American Pathology (CAP) certification. Also, by affording deep coverage, targeted panels enable detection of alterations in samples with low tumor purity or DNA content.

The majority of NGS assays and sequencing platforms are for research use only (RUO), with only a few, that is, MSK-IMPACT, FoundationOne CDx, and Guardant360 CDx, having received FDA approval (1). Therefore, implementation of a reliable clinical NGS assay in a diagnostic laboratory is crucial and requires extensive validation to establish CLIA- and CAP-compliant performance characteristics. For any laboratory developed test (LDT), the CLIA laboratory has to validate the designed testing sample types, assay performance, bioinformatic pipelines, variant interpretation, clinical reporting, data retrieval, and storage. The assay performance parameters include analytical sensitivity, analytical specificity, accuracy, precision, limit of detection, sequencing depth, and allelic frequency cutoffs (2).

Single-Nucleotide Polymorphism Microarray

Single-nucleotide polymorphism (SNP) microarray and microarray-based comparative genomic hybridization are high-throughput molecular technologies allowing genome-wide copy number profiling to detect actionable amplification and deletion. However, degradation of DNA derived from formalin-fixed paraffin-embedded (FFPE) tissue and the yield of DNA from solid tumors limit the use of many of these microarray assays for cancer genome analysis in clinical practice. In this respect, molecular inversion probe–based SNP microarray technology can work with DNA fragments as short as 40 bp and thus provide high-quality genomic data on CNAs in solid tumors including breast cancer when only nanograms of degraded DNA are extracted from FFPE tissue (3–5). In comparison with conventional FISH assay to detect *ERBB2(HER2)* amplification, molecular inversion probe–based SNP microarray can provide accurate and quantitative assessment of copy number gain/amplification and loss for nearly 900 cancer-related genes as well as copy-neutral loss of heterozygosity (LOH) of genes within chromosomal segments and chromothripsis (catastrophic event of massive chromosome shattering and complex genomic rearrangement involving localized regions of a single or a few chromosomes) (5–8).

RNA-Based Expression Profiling

RNA-based genomic expression profiling can provide predictive and prognostic signatures for the disease stratification of breast cancer patients (Table 2.1). The MammaPrint (70-gene, Agendia, Amsterdam, Netherlands) uses RNA microarray technology to predict the early distant recurrence within the first 5 years after diagnosis in estrogen receptor (ER)-positive or ER-negative breast cancer patients with primary tumor less than 5 cm (T1, T2) and lymph node–negative or –positive (0–3 nodes; N0, N1) disease (9,10). The Oncotype DX (21-gene, Exact Sciences, Madison, WI) and Endo-Predict (12-gene, Myriad Genetics Inc., Salt Lake City, UT) used quantitative RT-PCR (qRT-PCR) assay to test recurrence score in ER-positive primary breast cancer with N0 or N1 disease. The recurrence score predicts chemotherapy response in high-recurrence score group and the likelihood of distant recurrence in 10 years (11). EndoPredict provides late (5–10 years) distant recurrence after hormonal therapy (12). Prosigna (PAM50, 50-gene, NanoString Technologies, Seattle, WA) uses a qRT-PCR assay to test ER-positive or ER-negative primary breast cancer with stage I–III disease to provide intrinsic molecular subtypes (luminal A, luminal B, HER2 enriched and basal like) (13).

Oncotype DX is currently the only multigene panel listed as tier I by both the American Joint Committee on Cancer (AJCC) staging manual 8th edition and the National Comprehensive Cancer Network (NCCN) Guidelines V4.2021.

SAMPLE TESTING
Tumor Tissue Samples

Breast cancer specimens that are used for molecular diagnostics typically include routinely processed tissue samples collected for pathologic diagnosis. Specimens include histologic specimens in the form of a core needle biopsy and/or resection specimen, as well as cytologic specimens in the form of fine-needle aspirations and/or exfoliative specimens such as effusions with metastatic disease (Table 2.2). Most histologic specimens and a large fraction of cytologic specimens are routinely fixed in 10% neutral buffered formalin and embedded in low-melting-temperature paraffin to create a FFPE block that can be used to generate multiple serial sections for biomarker studies including IHC, FISH, and DNA/RNA-based molecular assays. In addition, tissue can also be procured as fresh, frozen samples as well as cytologic direct smear preparations and/or liquid-based cytology for specific molecular diagnostic studies; however, the use of any nonconventional substrate for molecular testing requires rigorous CLIA validation prior to any clinical use.

In general, the adequacy of any specimen for molecular diagnostics depends on (i) the overall cellularity of the sample that correlates with the DNA/RNA yield obtained for molecular testing and (ii) the tumor cellularity, which is the proportion of tumor cells relative to all nucleated cells contained within a specimen and determines the minimum acceptance criteria based on the analytical sensitivity (lowest limit of detection, LOD) of the molecular assay. For most practical purposes, the minimum tumor cellularity of a sample must be twice that of the analytical sensitivity of a molecular assay to be able to meet the LOD for reliably detecting mutant alleles in a tumor sample. For instance, NGS assays with an analytical sensitivity of 5% to 10% have a minimum tumor cellularity requirement of approximately 20% to avoid false-negative results.

Because gene expression profile assays are primarily RNA based, the quality of RNA retrieved from breast cancer specimens is critical. FFPE tissue has been shown to yield poor quality RNA compared with that obtained from frozen tissue because of chemical modifications and the partial degradation of the RNA, making RNA extraction, RT, and quantification more challenging.

Table 2.2 Sample Selection and Associated Preanalytic Factors for the Molecular Tests of Somatic Variants

Sample Type	Advantages	Limitations
Formalin-fixed paraffin-embedded (FFPE) tissue	• Standard for histologic evaluation for biopsy and excision • Long-term storage (in years) • Tumor fraction assessment • Tumor size and cellularity assessment • Tumor mapping to enrich tumor fraction • Viable tumor best for histologic evaluation and PCR-based sequencing • Nonviable tumor from apoptosis may be compatible with some PCR-based sequencing using short targeted sequences. • Bone lesion after decalcification with weak acid or EDTA compatible with some PCR-based sequencing	• DNA fragmentation due to formalin fixation • Nonviable or necrotic tumor from autolysis incompatible with PCR-based sequencing • Bone lesion after decalcification with strong acid not suitable for most PCR-based sequencing
Frozen tissue	• High-quality DNA • No formalin fixation artifact • Long-term storage at −80°C	• Presence of tumor in tissue and tumor fraction cannot be accurately evaluated.

Table 2.2 Sample Selection and Associated Preanalytic Factors for the Molecular Tests of Somatic Variants (*continued*)

Sample Type	Advantages	Limitations
Cytology smear	<ul><li>High-quality DNA</li><li>Immediate assessment</li><li>3-dimensional tumor clusters with intact nuclei</li><li>Air-dried methanol fixed, Diff-Quik stained or ethanol fixed, Papanicolaou (Pap) stained, no formalin fixation artifact</li><li>Ideal for metastatic and recurrent tumors</li></ul>	<ul><li>Inability to differentiate primary in situ versus invasive breast cancer</li><li>Requires sacrificing of the slide</li><li>Requires separate validation</li></ul>
Cytology cell blocks	<ul><li>Long-term storage (in years)</li><li>Tumor fraction assessment</li><li>Tumor cellularity assessment</li></ul>	<ul><li>No immediate assessment</li><li>DNA fragmentation due to formalin fixation</li><li>Inability to differentiate in situ versus invasive breast cancer</li></ul>
Body fluid and liquid-based preparations	<ul><li>High-quality DNA</li><li>Optimal preservation of nucleic acids</li></ul>	<ul><li>No immediate assessment</li></ul>
Circulating free DNA (cfDNA)	<ul><li>High-quality DNA</li><li>Noninvasive approach for detecting tumor-derived markers</li><li>cfDNA level correlates with tumor stages.</li></ul>	<ul><li>Low sensitivity with false-negative variant call in patients with early-stage cancer and without DNA release</li><li>No tumor fraction assessment</li></ul>

EDTA, ethylenediaminetetraacetic acid; PCR, polymerase chain reaction.

However, with FFPE tissue being the most widely available tissue specimen from routinely processed pathology specimens, most commercially available RNA-based molecular assays have been adequately validated for these specimens. Additional pre-analytical factors that impact nucleic acid quality such as necrosis, mucin, decalcification using harsh acids, heavy metal fixatives, and/or additives also affect molecular diagnostic testing success rates.

Normal Sample for Detecting Germline Mutations

Germline testing for breast cancer is typically performed on a peripheral blood or saliva sample that is collected into designated tubes/containers. Genetic consultation and patient consent are required for germline testing.

Normal Sample as Control for Detecting Somatic Variants

Some somatic NGS-based assays may require a normal control to distinguish somatic mutations from SNPs. Any normal sample including peripheral blood and benign tissue specimen with adequate cellularity can be used.

Tumor Types (Primary, Metastasis, Recurrence)

Genetic alterations are frequently correlated with specific tumor subtype, histology, and immuno-histochemical and molecular subtypes (Table 2.3) (14). The biomarker request should be specific for the tumor subtype and sample selection should be tailored for the specific molecular test. For example, *ESR1*, the gene that encodes for ERα, is exclusively present in ER-positive breast cancer. *ESR1* somatic mutations are present in approximately 25% to 30% of patients with metastatic/recurrent ER-positive breast cancer who received hormonal therapies, especially in those who received aromatase inhibitors (15–18). *ESR1* is significantly mutated in metastatic breast cancer (~20%) as compared to primary breast cancer (<1%) (15,19). Therefore, biomarker testing for *ESR1* somatic mutation should target ER-positive (not ER-negative) breast cancer patients with distant metastasis or recurrent diseases. In general, when NGS assay is performed to detect somatic variants in advanced breast cancer patients, the tumor samples from most recent recurrent/

metastatic site are preferable because the therapy is targeted to current recurrent tumor, not the previously excised primary tumor. The multigene expression profiles such as Oncotype DX are send-out assays performed at commercial laboratories to provide predictive and prognostic values for primary breast cancer patients. These RNA-based assays were validated in primary tumors and therefore primary tumors (not lymph node metastasis) should be used.

Circulating Free DNA

There has been an increasing use of liquid biopsy in the realm of solid tumor malignancies, especially in patients with insufficient tumor tissue for molecular profiling and/or to monitor treatment response and resistance mechanisms. The two main types of liquid biopsies utilized clinically include circulating free DNA (cfDNA) and circulating tumor cells (CTCs). cfDNA are small DNA fragments (around 160 bp) that are shed by the tumor (circulating tumor DNA) into the blood stream, whereas CTCs are intact tumor cells in the blood stream. cfDNA is more abundant in the peripheral blood than CTCs, and therefore, current commercially available liquid biopsy assays are focused mostly on plasma-based cfDNA. Specimens are collected in ethylenediaminetetraacetic acid (EDTA), heparin, and specialized blood collection tubes such as Streck tubes that contain a preservative stabilizing nucleated blood cells. The stabilization agent prevents the release of genomic DNA and allows isolation of high-quality cfDNA.

ACTIONABLE GENETIC ALTERATIONS AND PATHWAYS IN BREAST CANCER

The actionable breast cancer–relevant signaling pathways and their associated genetic alterations are summarized in Table 2.3. In hormonal signaling pathway, the recurrent gain-of-function *ESR1* somatic mutations have been reported in approximately 20% of patients with metastatic ER-positive breast cancer who received hormonal therapies, especially in those who received aromatase inhibitors (15–18). The recurrent *ESR1* fusions, relatively rare (<1%), have also been implicated for hormonal therapy resistance (20). In cell surface (transmembrane) receptors, the HER2 overexpression and/or amplification, present in approximately 20% of breast cancers, are associated with aggressive clinical course, but predict a better response to anti-HER2 therapy. *HER2* somatic mutations have been reported in approximately 2% of breast cancers in both ductal and lobular carcinoma (21).

Table 2.3 Overview of Clinically Relevant Genetic Alterations in Breast Cancer

Gene	Cytoband	Protein	Aberration
AKT1	14q32.33	AKT serine/threonine kinase 1	Activating mutation
AKT3	1q44	AKT serine/threonine kinase 3	Activating mutation
*ATM**	11q22.3	ATM serine/threonine kinase	Loss-of-function mutation
*BRCA1**	17q21.31	Breast cancer type 1 susceptibility protein	Loss-of-function mutation
*BRCA2**	13q13.1	Breast cancer type 2 susceptibility protein	Loss-of-function mutation
*BRIP1**	17q23.2	BRCA1 interacting protein C-terminal helicase 1	Loss-of-function mutation
*CDH1**	16q22.1	E-cadherin (cadherin-1)	Loss of expression
			Loss-of-function mutation
*CHEK2**	22q12.1	Checkpoint kinase 2	Loss-of-function mutation

Testing Assays	Pathway	Subgroup Association	Implications for Targeted Therapeutics
DNA sequencing	PI3K pathway	Metastatic	PI3K inhibitor, AKT inhibitor
DNA sequencing	PI3K pathway	None	AKT inhibitor
DNA sequencing	DNA damage response	ER positive	Radiation therapy may be contraindicated
DNA sequencing	Cell cycle, DNA repair	High grade, "medullary like," triple negative	PARP inhibitor
DNA sequencing	Cell cycle, DNA repair	None	PARP inhibitor
DNA sequencing	DNA repair	None	PARP inhibitor
IHC	Cell adhesion	Lobular	ROS1 inhibitor
DNA sequencing			
DNA sequencing	DNA damage response	ER positive	PARP inhibitor

(continued)

Table 2.3 Overview of Clinically Relevant Genetic Alterations in Breast Cancer (continued)

Gene	Cytoband	Protein	Aberration
ESR1	6q25.1-q25.2	Estrogen receptor-α	Protein expression
			Activating mutation
			Translocation
HER2 (ERBB2)	17q12	Erb-b2 receptor tyrosine kinase 2 (HER2)	Protein expression
			Protein/RNA overexpression
			Gene amplification
			Activating mutation
NBN*	8q21.3	Nibrin	Loss-of-function mutation
NF1*	17q11.2	Neurofibromin 1	Loss-of-function mutation
NTRK3	15q25.3	Neurotrophic receptor tyrosine kinase 3	Translocation

Testing Assays	Pathway	Subgroup Association	Implications for Targeted Therapeutics
IHC	Hormone signaling pathway	Metastatic ER positive	Acquired resistance to endocrine therapy in ER-positive aromatase inhibitor–treated metastatic breast cancer
DNA sequencing			
RNA fusion assay			
IHC	EGFR pathway		Sensitive to anti-HER2 antibody drug conjugate
IHC, RNA expression		Apocrine features	Sensitive to anti-HER2 therapies
FISH, SNP microarray, NGS			
DNA sequencing		High-grade lobular, or metastatic *HER2* amplified	Anti-HER2 therapy
DNA sequencing	Cell cycle, DNA damage, DNA repair	None	PARP inhibitors
DNA sequencing	GTPase activation	None	mTOR inhibitors
IHC, FISH, RNA fusion assay	PI3K and MAPK pathways	Secretory breast carcinoma	TRK inhibitor

(continued)

Table 2.3 Overview of Clinically Relevant Genetic Alterations in Breast Cancer (continued)

Gene	Cytoband	Protein	Aberration
PALB2*	16p12.2	Partner and localizer of BRCA2	Loss-of-function mutation
PIK3CA	3q26.32	PI3-kinase p110 subunit α	Activating mutation
PTEN*	10q23.31	Phosphatase and tensin homolog (PTEN)	Protein loss
			Gene deletion
			Loss-of-function mutation
RET	10q11.21	Ret proto-oncogene	Fusion
TP53*	17p13.1	Tumor protein p53	Loss-of-function mutation

Testing Assays	Pathway	Subgroup Association	Implications for Targeted Therapeutics
DNA sequencing	DNA repair	None	PARP inhibitor
DNA sequencing	PI3K pathway	Metastatic or lobular	PI3K inhibitor
IHC	PI3K pathways	Lobular or metastatic	PI3K inhibitor
DNA sequencing			PARP inhibitor
FISH, RNA fusion assay	PI3K and MAPK pathways	None	RET inhibitor
DNA sequencing	Cell cycle, DNA repair	Triple negative, HER2 positive, or metastatic	Resistance to DNA-damaging chemo agents

ER, estrogen receptor; FISH, fluorescence in situ hybridization; IHC, immunohistochemistry; MAPK, mitogen-activated protein kinase; NGS, next-generation sequencing; PARP, poly(ADP-ribose) polymerase; PI3K, phosphatidylinositol 3-kinase; SNP, single-nucleotide polymorphism; TRK, tropomyosin receptor kinase.
*Germline mutation associated with hereditary breast cancer: BRCA1/2 in hereditary breast/ovarian cancer, CDH1 in hereditary diffuse gastric cancer and lobular breast cancer, PTEN in Cowden syndrome, and TP3 in Li–Fraumeni syndrome

The *ETV6–NTRK3* fusion defines a rare histologic subtype, secretory breast carcinoma (22–24). The neurotrophic receptor tyrosine kinase (NTRK) inhibitor approved by the FDA for the treatment of unresectable or metastatic solid tumors bearing NTRK fusions also works for secretory breast carcinoma (25–27). The phosphatidylinositol 3-kinase (PI3K) pathway genes *PIK3CA* and *AKT1* are frequently mutated in ER-positive breast cancer, 43% and 3%, respectively (14). The phosphatase and tensin homolog (PTEN) negatively regulates PI3K signaling pathway. PTEN somatic mutations (7%) and deletions (6%) are mutually exclusive with *PIK3CA* somatic mutations (28). Multiple PI3K inhibitors are under investigation and have shown survival benefit in patients with PIK3CA-mutated or PTEN-mutated tumors (29–33). In cell cycle and DNA repair pathway, the BReast CAncer genes *BRCA1* (17q21.31) and *BRCA2* (13q13.1) are parts of a homologous recombination complex playing important role in repairing double-strand DNA breaks during cell cycle (34). Inhibitors of poly(ADP-ribose) polymerase (PARP), an enzyme involved in single-strand DNA break repair, have been approved by the FDA for treating advanced breast cancer patients with germline *BRCA1 or BRCA2* mutation. Currently, investigational clinical trials are exploring the clinical utility of PARP inhibitors in metastatic breast cancer patients with either germline or somatic mutations in DNA repair genes (*BRCA1*, *BRCA2*, and other homologous recombination deficiency [HRD] genes).

FoundationOne CDx

FoundationOne CDx is a NGS-based diagnostic test that uses targeted high-throughput hybridization-based capture technology for the detection of substitutions, indels, rearrangements, and CNVs in 324 genes (309 cancer-related genes, 1 promoter region, 1 noncoding [ncRNA], and select intronic regions from 34 commonly rearranged genes, 21 of which also include the coding exons) as well as genomic signatures including MSI and TMB using DNA isolated from FFPE tissue specimens. The test is intended as a companion diagnostic to identify patients who may benefit from treatment with the FDA-approved targeted therapies as listed in Table 2.4.

FoundationOne Liquid CDx is a qualitative NGS diagnostic test that uses targeted high-throughput hybridization-based capture technology to detect substitutions, indels in 311 genes, rearrangements in 4 genes, and CNAs in 3 genes. It uses cfDNA isolated from plasma derived from anticoagulated peripheral whole blood. The test is intended as a companion diagnostic to identify patients who may benefit from treatment with the FDA-approved targeted therapies as listed in Table 2.5. Patients with the tumor types listed earlier who are negative for the mutations listed later should be reflexed to routine biopsy and their tumor mutation status confirmed using an FDA-approved tumor tissue NGS assay.

GUARDANT360

Guardant360 CDx is a qualitative NGS-based in vitro diagnostic device that uses targeted high-throughput hybridization-based capture technology for the detection of SNVs, indels in 55 genes, CNAs in 2 genes, and fusions in 4 genes frequently altered in cancers. It utilizes cfDNA from plasma of peripheral whole blood collected in Streck cfDNA Blood Collection Tubes. It is intended to be used as a companion diagnostic to identify non–small cell lung cancer (NSCLC) patients who may benefit from treatment with the targeted therapies listed in Table 2.6 in accordance with the approved therapeutic product labeling.

Table 2.4 Diagnostic Indications for FoundationOne CDx

Tumor Type	Biomarker	Targeted Therapy
Breast cancer	*ERBB2 (HER2)* amplification	Trastuzumab, Pertuzumab, T-DM1
	PIK3CA C420R, E542K, E545A, E545D [1635G>T only], E545G, E545K, Q546E, Q546R, H1047L, H1047R, and H1047Y alterations	Alpelisib
Colorectal cancer	*KRAS* wild type (absence of mutations in codons 12 and 13)	Cetuximab
	KRAS wild type (absence of mutations in exons 2, 3, and 4) and *NRAS* wild type (absence of mutations in exons 2, 3, and 4)	Panitumumab
Cholangiocarcinoma	*FGFR2* fusions and select rearrangements	Pemigatinib, Infigratinib
Melanoma	*BRAF* V600E	FDA-approved BRAF inhibitors
	BRAF V600E and V600K	Trametinib or FDA-approved BRAF/MEK inhibitor combinations

Table 2.4 Diagnostic Indications for FoundationOne CDx (*continued*)

Tumor Type	Biomarker	Targeted Therapy
Non–small cell lung cancer	*EGFR* exon 19 deletions and *EGFR* exon 21 L858R alterations	Afatinib, Gefitinib, Osimertinib, Erlotinib
	EGFR exon 20 T790M alterations	Osimertinib
	ALK rearrangements	Alectinib, Brigatinib, Crizotinib, Ceritinib
	BRAF V600E	Dabrafenib with Trametinib
	MET single-nucleotide variants (SNVs) and indels that lead to MET exon 14 skipping	Capmatinib
Ovarian cancer	*BRCA1/2* alterations	Olaparib, Rucaparib
Prostate cancer	Homologous Recombination Repair (HRR) gene (*BRCA1, BRCA2, ATM, BARD1, BRIP1, CDK12, CHEK1, CHEK2, FANCL, PALB2, RAD51B, RAD51C, RAD51D,* and *RAD54L*) alterations	Olaparib
Solid tumors	TMB ≥10 mutations per Mb	Pembrolizumab
	NTRK1/2/3 fusions	Larotrectinib

Table 2.5 Diagnostic Indications for FoundationOne Liquid CDx

Tumor Type	Biomarker	Targeted Therapy
Breast cancer	*PIK3CA* C420R, E542K, E545A, E545D [1635G>T only], E545G, E545K, Q546E, Q546R, H1047L, H1047R, and H1047Y mutations	Alpelisib
Non–small cell lung cancer	*EGFR* exon 19 deletions and *EGFR* exon 21 L858R substitutions	Gefitinib, Osimertinib, Erlotinib
	ALK rearrangements	Alectinib
	MET single-nucleotide variants (SNVs) and indels that lead to MET exon 14 skipping	Capmatinib
Ovarian cancer	*BRCA1/2* alterations	Rucaparib
Prostate cancer	*BRCA1*, *BRCA2*, *ATM* alterations	Olaparib
	BRCA1, *BRCA2* alterations	Rucaparib

MSK-IMPACT

MSK-IMPACT (integrated mutation profiling of actionable cancer targets) is a qualitative in vitro diagnostic test that uses targeted NGS of FFPE tumor tissue matched with normal specimens from patients with solid malignant neoplasms to detect SNVs, indels, and MSI in 468 cancer-associated genes. The test is intended to provide information on somatic mutations (point mutations and small insertions and deletions) and MSI for clinical use; however, it is not conclusive or prescriptive for labeled use of any specific therapeutic product.

Table 2.6 Diagnostic Indications for Guardant360 CDx

Tumor Type	Biomarker	Targeted Therapy
Non–small cell lung cancer	*EGFR exon 19 deletions, L858R and T790M**	Osimertinib
	EGFR exon 20 insertions	Amivantamab
	KRAS G12C	Sotorasib

*Indicated for whom tumor biopsy cannot be obtained.

CARIS

CARIS provides comprehensive molecular testing to assess alterations in DNA, RNA, as well as protein expression. WES analyses of DNA for SNVs, CNVs, indels, LOH, MSI, TMB, as well as transcriptome analysis to identify fusions are performed across tumors.

Tempus

Tempus xT NGS assay covers 648 genes to detect SNVs, indels, CNVs, and translocations along with two promoter regions (PMS2 and TERT) and 239 sites to determine MSI status. RNA-Seq is also used to report gene fusions. For solid tumors, an FFPE tumor sample is sequenced along with a matched normal blood or saliva sample (when available). Clinical sequencing is performed to 500× depth of coverage for tumor specimens and 150× for normal specimens.

Tempus xF liquid biopsy assay detects cfDNA in blood specimens of advanced solid tumor patients. The assay can detect alterations in 105 genes including SNVs, indels, as well as CNV in 6 genes, copy number deletions in 2 genes (*BRCA1/2*), and gene rearrangements in 7 genes. MSI-High (MSI-H) status is also reported. The assay requires two 8.5 mL Streck tubes of peripheral blood with sequencing performed to ~20,000× coverage (at least 5,000× deduplicated reads).

FDA-Approved Companion Diagnostics in Breast and Other Solid Tumors

Test	Vendor	Indication for Tumor Type	Agent
BRACAnalysis CDx	Myriad	Breast cancer	Olaparib Talazoparib
		Ovarian cancer	Olaparib Rucaparib
		Pancreatic cancer	Olaparib
		CRPC	Olaparib
Therascreen PIK3CA RGQ PCR Kit	Qiagen	Breast cancer	Alpelisib
Ki-67 IHC MIB-1 pharmDx (Dako Omnis)	Agilent	Breast cancer	Abemaciclib
FoundationOne CDx	Foundation Medicine	Breast cancer	Trastuzumab Pertuzumab T-DM1 Alpelisib
		Solid tumors (TMB ≥10 mutations per Mb)	Pembrolizumab
		Solid tumors (NTRK1/2/3 fusions)	Larotrectinib

Test	Vendor	Indication for Tumor Type	Agent
		NSCLC	Afatinib Gefitinib Erlotinib Osimertinib Alectinib Brigatinib Crizotinib Ceritinib Dabrafenib with Trametinib Capmatinib
		Melanoma	Dabrafenib Vemurafenib Trametinib with Vemurafenib Cobimetinib with Vemurafenib Encorafenib with Binimetinib
		Colorectal cancer	Cetuximab Panitumumab
		Ovarian cancer	Rucaparib Olaparib

(*continued*)

Test	Vendor	Indication for Tumor Type	Agent
		Cholangiocarcinoma	Pemigatinib Infigratinib
		CRPC	Olaparib
PD-L1 22C3 Assay	Dako	TNBC NSCLC Gastric/GEJ tumor Cervical cancer Urothelial cancer HNSCC ESCC	Pembrolizumab Cemiplimab
PD-L1 SP142 Assay	Ventana	TNBC Urothelial cancer NSCLC	Atezolizumab
VENTANA MMR RxDx Panel	Ventana	Mismatch repair deficient (dMMR) solid tumors Endometrial carcinoma	Dostarlimab
INFORM HER-2/neu	Ventana	Breast cancer	Trastuzumab T-DM1
PathVysion HER-2 DNA Probe Kit	Abbott	Breast cancer	Trastuzumab

Test	Vendor	Indication for Tumor Type	Agent
PATHWAY anti-Her2/neu (4B5) Antibody	Ventana	Breast cancer	Trastuzumab T-DM1
InSite Her-2/neu KIT	Biogenex	Breast cancer	Trastuzumab
SPOT-LIGHT HER2 CISH Kit	Life Technologies	Breast cancer	Trastuzumab
Bond Oracle HER2 IHC System	Leica	Breast cancer	Trastuzumab
HER2 CISH pharmDx Kit	Dako	Breast cancer	Trastuzumab
HercepTest	Dako	Breast cancer	Trastuzumab Pertuzumab T-DM1
		Gastric/gastroesophageal cancer	Trastuzumab
HER2 FISH pharmDx Kit	Dako	Breast cancer	Trastuzumab Pertuzumab T-DM1
		Gastric/gastroesophageal cancer	Trastuzumab

(*continued*)

Test	Vendor	Indication for Tumor Type	Agent
Therascreen EGFR PCR Kit	Qiagen	NSCLC	Gefitinib Afatinib Dacomitinib
Cobas EGFR Mutation Test V2	Roche	NSCLC	Tissue Erlotinib Osimertinib Gefitinib Afatinib Dacomitinib Plasma Erlotinib Osimertinib Gefitinib
ALK D5F3 CDx	Ventana	NSCLC	Ceritinib Crizotinib Alectinib Lorlatinib
Oncomine Dx Target Test	Life Technologies	NSCLC	Gefitinib Crizotinib Pralsetinib Mobocertinib Dabrafenib with Trametinib
		Cholangiocarcinoma	Ivosidenib

Test	Vendor	Indication for Tumor Type	Agent
Therascreen KRAS RGQ PCR Kit	Qiagen	NSCLC Colorectal cancer	Sotorasib Cetuximab Panitumumab
Vysis ALK FISH Kit	Abbott	NSCLC	Crizotinib Brigatinib
ONCO/Reveal Dx Lung and Colon Cancer Assay (O/RDx-LCCA)	Pillar Biosciences	NSCLC Colorectal	Gefitinib Afatinib Erlotinib Dacomitinib Cetuximab Panitumumab
PD-L1 28-8 Assay	Dako	NSCLC	Nivolumab with Ipilimumab
PD-L1 SP263 Assay	Ventana	NSCLC	Atezolizumab
Cobas KRAS Mutation Test	Roche	Colorectal cancer	Cetuximab Panitumumab
Praxis RAS Panel	Illumina	Colon cancer	Panitumumab
Dako EGFR pharmDx	Dako	Colorectal cancer	Cetuximab Panitumumab

(*continued*)

Test	Vendor	Indication for Tumor Type	Agent
Therascreen BRAF V600E RGQ PCR Kit	Qiagen	Colorectal cancer	Encorafenib with Cetuximab
FoundationFocus CDx BRCA Assay	Foundation Medicine	Ovarian cancer	Rucaparib
Myriad myChoice CDx	Myriad	Ovarian cancer	Niraparib Olaparib
THXID BRAF Kit	bioMerieux	Melanoma	Trametinib Dabrafenib Encorafenib with Binimetinib
cobas 4800 BRAF V600 Mutation Test	Roche	Melanoma	Vemurafenib Cobimetinib with Vemurafenib
Therascreen FGFR RGQ RT-PCR Kit	Qiagen	Urothelial cancer	Erdafitinib
Dako c-KIT pharmDx	Dako	GIST	Imatinib

FoundationOne Liquid CDx	Foundation Medicine	**Breast cancer**	Alpelisib
		NSCLC	Gefitinib Osimertinib Erlotinib Alectinib Capmatinib
		CRPC	Rucaparib Olaparib
		Ovarian cancer	Rucaparib
Guardant360 CDx	Guardant Health	NSCLC	Osimertinib Amivantamab Sotorasib

CISH, chromogenic in situ hybridization; CRPC, castrate-resistant prostate cancer; EGFR, epidermal growth factor receptor; ESCC, esophageal squamous cell cancer; FDA, Food and Drug Administration; FISH, fluorescence in situ hybridization; GEJ, gastroesophageal junction; GIST, gastrointestinal stromal tumors; HNSCC, head and neck squamous cell cancer; IHC, immunohistochemistry; NSCLC, non–small cell lung cancer; PCR, polymerase chain reaction; PD-L1, Programmed death-ligand 1; TMB, tumor mutational burden; TNBC, triple-negative breast cancer. For the most current information about the FDA-approved companion diagnostics, go to: https://www.fda.gov/medical-devices/in-vitro-diagnostics/list-cleared-or-approved-companion-diagnostic-devices-in-vitro-and-imaging-tools.

SOMATIC AND GERMLINE VARIANT IDENTIFICATION

Because clinical tumor testing primarily utilizes targeted gene panels that focus on known mutational hotspots, paired germline DNA testing is typically not performed.

Although the matched normal-tumor DNA analysis provides the most optimal approach in differentiating a germline from somatic mutation, this is not widely employed in clinical practice because of logistical issues (35). Nevertheless, it is important to recognize that germline alterations can be identified based on tumor-only sequencing, even without analysis of germline DNA. Alteration in genes such as *BRCA1/2*, *PALB2* also has therapeutic implications. Incidental pathogenic germline variants (PGVs) have been reported in approximately 5% of patients who underwent targeted gene panel testing (36).

There are a few scenarios when a germline variant can be inferred from tumor-only sequencing. The most common scenario is when the gene has been described to have both somatic and germline variants as part of cancer susceptibility syndromes. These include genes such as *VHL* or *TP53* (Table 2.7). In such cases, to discern somatic variants from germline, it is important to consider the patient's age, tumor type, personal history of cancers, and a detailed family history. For example, *VHL* mutation observed in a tumor gene panel in a 40-year-old patient with bilateral renal carcinoma associated with pheochromocytoma and retinal hemangioblastoma is likely to represent a germline variant, whereas a *VHL* mutation observed with tumor-only sequencing in a 65-year-old is likely to be somatic. Specific mutational patterns can also suggest an underlying germline mutation. For example, chromothripsis (clustered genomic rearrangements and deletions involving one or more chromosomes) is highly suggestive of an underlying germline mutation in *TP53* (37). A hypermutated pattern could suggest an underlying germline mutation in *POLE* and *POLD1* DNA polymerases or DNA mismatch repair genes (38–40). Clinical tumor sequencing can also recognize mutations in specific genes that are highly indicative of a germline variant. For example, identification of founder mutations in *BRCA1* (185 delAG) or *BRCA2* (6174delT and 5382insC) in tumor gene panels likely suggests an underlying germline defect.

Table 2.7 Gene Alterations That Are Indicative of Potential Pathogenic Germline Variants

APC	CHEK2	NF1	STK11
ATM	EPCAM	PALB2	TSC2
BRCA1	FANC	PMS2	TP53
BRCA2	MLH1	PTEN	VHL
BRIP1	MSH2	RAD51C	
CDKN2A	MSH6	RAD51D	
CDK1	NBN	RB1	

Inherited cancer syndromes mediated by germline mutations tend to have early age on onset, associated with specific tumor types and strong personal or family history of cancers (Table 2.8). Also, PGVs tend to be SNVs or small deletions or insertions and are seldom due to translocations (41). Importantly, because DNA from tumors are often admixed with normal tissue, variant allele fraction (VAF) can potentially indicate a germline versus somatic alteration. VAF is the fraction of mutant allele in the sample (or the expected fraction of supporting reads) and is dependent on tumor purity and cancer cell fraction. Germline mutations tend to have VAF close to 50% for heterozygous or 100% for homozygous variants. Whereas the allele fraction for somatic mutation tends to be lower because of normal tissue contamination, this approach cannot reliably identify germline from somatic alterations if the tumor cellularity is greater than 50% (42).

Table 2.8 Features That Can Be Used to Discern a Somatic from Germline Variant

Age
Tumor type
Personal history of cancers
Family history
Type of alteration
Variant allele fraction
Identical mutation occurring independently in two separate tumors

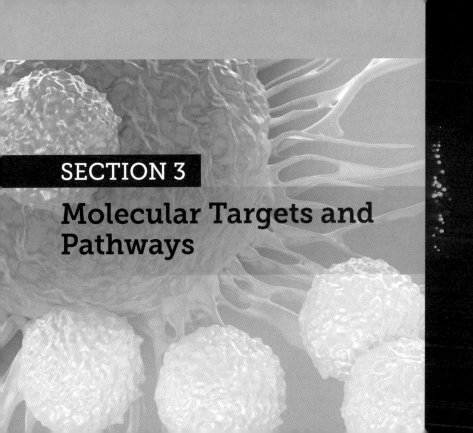

SECTION 3

Molecular Targets and Pathways

It is hard to do justice to the exquisite complexity of the cancer cell and to help comprehend the level of intra- and intercell signaling that occurs in the billions of cells in the human body. We have attempted to create an "org chart" to help classify the targets and strategies used to develop precision cancer treatment. There are three broad categories:

A. **Membrane Factors and Receptors (M 1–7)**: Receptor Tyrosine Kinases (RTKs) for Survival Factors, Chemokines and Transmitters, and Growth Factors, the Extracellular Matrix, Fruit Fly Mutations, Death Receptors (DRs), and Cytokine Receptors

B. **Intracellular Systems (1–10)**: Rapamycin, NF-Kappa B, G-Coupled Proteins, Mitogen-Activated Protein (MAP) Kinase (MAPK), SRC, β-Catenin, Caspases, Janus Kinase/Signal Transducer and Transcription (JAK/STAT), and Apoptosis

C. **Nuclear Factors, Cell Cycle Control, and DNA Repair (N)**: MYC, Extracellular Signal–Regulated Kinase (ERK), Cyclins, Retinoblastoma (RB), MDM2, TP53

COLOR KEY

 Agonist

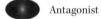 Antagonist

Signal Transduction Roadmap

M1	Survival Factors/VEGF	C6	β-Catenin/APC
M2	Chemokines/Hormones	C7	Cell Regulators
M3	Growth Factors	C8	Caspases/BCL2
M4	Extracellular Matrix	C9	JAK/STAT
M5	Fruit Fly Receptors	C10	Apoptosis
M6	Death Receptors	N1	Extracell. Reg. Kinases
M7	Cytokines/Interleukins	N2	Cyclins
C1	Rapamycin/mTOR Sys	N3	Retinoblastoma/RB
C2	NF-Kappa B	N4	MYC
C3	G-Proteins/Cyclic AMP	N5	MDM2
C4	RAS→RAF→MAPKinase	N6	TP53/DNA Repair
C5	Sarcoma Gene—SRC	N7	Other Nuclear Factors

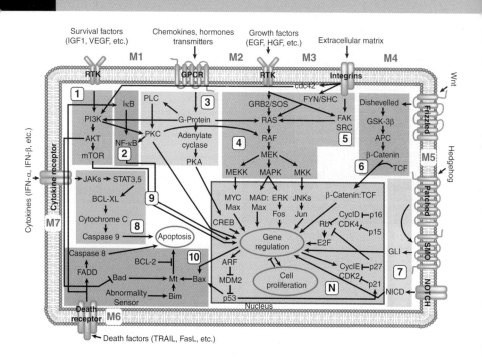

- Vascular endothelial growth factor (VEGF) is one of the most important and prominent proangiogenic factors. VEGF's normal function is to create new blood vessels during embryonic development, new blood vessels after injury, muscle following exercise, and new vessels (collateral circulation) to bypass blocked vessels.
- The VEGF family consists of five members (VEGF-A, -B, -C, -D, and placental growth factor [PlGF]), which transmit signals via three VEGF receptors (VEGFR-1 through VEGFR-3).
- Many human cancers are found to overexpress VEGFs and/or VEGFRs.
  - VEGFR-1 binding by VEGF-B plays a role in the maintenance of newly formed blood vessels.
  - VEGFR-2 activation by VEGF-A binding has been shown to stimulate endothelial cell (EC) mitogenesis and cell migration, leading to cancer progression and metastasis.
  - VEGFR-3 is predominantly expressed in lymphatic vessels. When bound by either VEGF-C or VEGF-D, VEGFR-3 plays a role in lymphangiogenesis and metastatic spread to lymph nodes in a pathologic setting.

Physiology	VEGF-A, -B, -C, -D and PlGF activate VEGFR-1, -2, -3 to promote vascularization
	• during embryogenesis • after injury • after vessel blockage • after exercise
Oncogenic VEGF, VEGFR behaviors	• Overexpressed in many cancers; expression associated with invasiveness, recurrence, prognosis • R2 activation by VEGF-A drives EC division and migration, and thus angiogenesis, cancer progression, metastasis. • R3 activation by VEGF-C, -D promotes metastasis to lymph nodes.

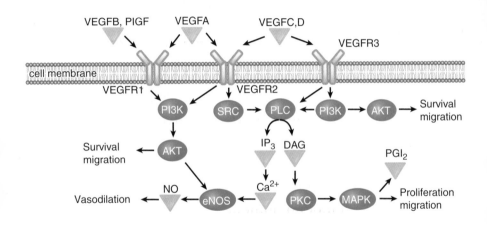

- Fibroblast growth factor receptor (FGFR) family has four highly conserved transmembrane RTKs (FGFR1–4) that differ in their ligand affinities and tissue distribution.
- Fibroblast growth factors (FGFs) include 18 structurally related polypeptides (FGF1–10, FGF16–23) that signal through FGFRs.
- FGFRs can bind canonical FGFs that are in complex with heparan sulfate proteoglycans (HSPGs) in an autocrine and paracrine fashion.
- FGFRs can also bind endocrine FGFs (FGF19, 21, and 23) that are found in circulation, free of HSPGs.
- Once bound to their ligands, FGFRs are induced to dimerize and cross-phosphorylate the tyrosine kinase domain on the cognate receptor.
- Various downstream effector molecules are then recruited, allowing for the activation of signaling events that culminate in regulation of various cellular processes such as cell survival and proliferation, organ development, angiogenesis, and tissue homeostasis, to name a few.
- Each FGFR can be activated by several FGFs; conversely, FGFs can activate more than one receptor.
- Dysregulation of FGFR signaling in cancer may be caused by the following:
  ○ *FGFR* gene amplifications, activating mutations, translocations, and fusions
  ○ Amplification of FGF and FGF-related genes
- Dysregulated FGFR signaling may contribute to cancer by the following:
  ○ Stimulating cancer cell proliferation
  ○ Driving tumor neovascularization
  ○ Promoting resistance to anticancer therapies

PHYSIOLOGY

- FGF1–10, FGF16–23 regulate essential cellular processes via FGFR1–4.
- Canonical FGFs elicit paracrine and autocrine effects.
- Others (FGF19, 21, 23) elicit endocrine effects.
- An FGF can trigger multiple FGFRs; an FGFR may engage several FGFs.
- Dysregulated signaling may promote cancer cell proliferation, tumor vascularization, and drug resistance.

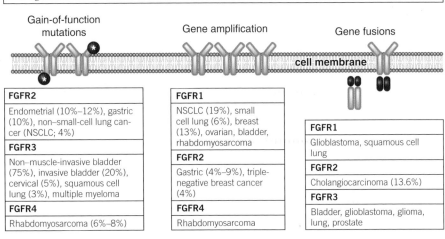

Gain-of-function mutations

Gene amplification

Gene fusions

cell membrane

FGFR2
Endometrial (10%–12%), gastric (10%), non–small-cell lung cancer (NSCLC; 4%)

FGFR3
Non–muscle-invasive bladder (75%), invasive bladder (20%), cervical (5%), squamous cell lung (3%), multiple myeloma

FGFR4
Rhabdomyosarcoma (6%–8%)

FGFR1
NSCLC (19%), small cell lung (6%), breast (13%), ovarian, bladder, rhabdomyosarcoma

FGFR2
Gastric (4%–9%), triple-negative breast cancer (4%)

FGFR4
Rhabdomyosarcoma

FGFR1
Glioblastoma, squamous cell lung

FGFR2
Cholangiocarcinoma (13.6%)

FGFR3
Bladder, glioblastoma, glioma, lung, prostate

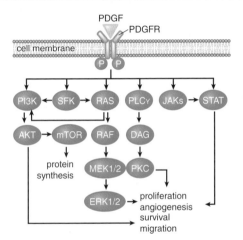

PHYSIOLOGY

- Platelet-derived growth factor (PDGF) A–D are potent mitogens for cells of mesenchymal origin.
- Synthesized, stored, and released by platelets upon activation
- Also produced by smooth muscle cells, activated macrophages, and ECs
- Essential in early development, tissue remodeling, differentiation
- Downstream effector pathways (MAPK, phosphatidylinositol 3-kinase [PI3K], and/or JAK/STAT) are triggered via PDGF receptor (PDGFR)A, B.

ONCOLOGIC BEHAVIORS

- *COL1A1–PDGFB* fusion linked to dermatofibrosarcoma protuberans
- PDGFRA mutations linked to multiple tumor types; germline lesions linked to hereditary gastrointestinal stromal tumors (GIST)
- *PDGFRA* amplification often associated with coalterations in epidermal growth factor receptor (*EGFR*), *KIT*, *KDR*
- Up to 60% of PDGFRA mutant GIST are also D842V, which is associated with primary resistance.

- PDGFs are potent mitogens for cells of mesenchymal origin and are synthesized, stored, and released by platelets upon activation; also produced by smooth muscle cells, activated macrophages, and ECs.
- PDGF signaling network consists of four ligands (PDGFA–D) and two transmembrane tyrosine RTKs (PDGFRα and PDGFRβ).
- These receptors transmit extracellular growth factor signaling to intracellular signaling cascades. Upon binding of the growth factor ligands, the receptors undergo dimerization and autophosphorylation of cytoplasmic kinase domains, activating the receptor.
- Downstream effects of PDGFR activation lead to differential signaling through MAPK, PI3K, and/or JAK/STAT pathways, resulting in cell proliferation, cell differentiation, survival, and migration.
- Dermatofibrosarcoma protuberans is characterized by a chromosomal translocation with formation of COL1A1–PDGFB fusion gene, causing activation of PDGFRβ in tumor cells.
- PDGFRα is encoded by the *PDGFRA* gene, which is altered in multiple tumor types, resulting in constitutive PDGFRα activity.
- Germline mutations in PDGFRA have been described in hereditary GIST.
- PDGFRA amplification has been described in sarcomas and gliomas; however, often it is associated with coalterations in EGFR, KIT, and KDR.
- In about 5% of GIST, somatic PDGFRA mutations in exons 12, 14, and 18 activation loop are the most common and are associated with greater response to PDGFRA-inhibitor imatinib. However, up to 60% of PDGFRA mutant GIST harbors a mutation in exon 18 D842V, which is associated with primary resistance.

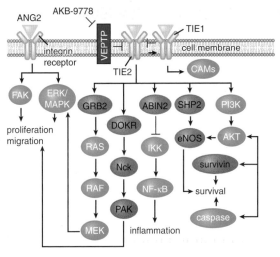

PHYSIOLOGY

- Angiopoietin growth factors (ANG) regulate angiogenesis through activating (ANG1,4) or inhibitory (ANG2,3) effects on TIE1,2.
- ANG-TIE system is critical for cardiac, blood, vascular development and homeostasis.

ASSOCIATED PATHOLOGIC STATES

- inflammation
- metastasis
- tumor angiogenesis
- atherosclerosis
- vascular leakage

ONCOGENIC BEHAVIORS

- Circulating ANG2 predictive of poor prognosis from many cancers
- Low baseline ANG2 predicts better response to anti-VEGF therapy versus colorectal cancer.
- High baseline serum ANG2 predicts poorer outcome from immune checkpoint therapy; potentially immunosuppressive.
- ANG bind to cell surface RTKs with immunoglobulin-like and epithelial growth factor–like domains 1 and 2 (TIE1 and TIE2).
- Four different ANGs have been identified (ANG1, ANG2, ANG3, and ANG4).
- ANG1 and ANG4 are agonists for TIE2, whereas ANG2 and ANG3 are competitive antagonists for TIE1 and TIE2.
- Activation of TIE2 by ANG1 is indispensable for embryonic cardiac development and angiogenesis, and both TIE1 and TIE2 are key regulators of normal formation of blood and lymphatic vessel development as TIE1 and TIE2 are almost exclusively expressed in the endothelium.
- ANG/TIE system is also involved in pathologic processes including inflammation, metastasis, tumor angiogenesis, atherosclerosis, and vascular leakage.
- Upon binding of ANG ligands, TIE2 receptors can form dimers or possibly multimers. Vascular endothelial protein tyrosine phosphatase (VEPTP, encoded by *PTPRB* gene) dephosphorylates active TIE2.
- TIE1 upregulates the cell adhesion molecules (CAMs) VCAM-1, E-selectin, and ICAM-1 through a p38-dependent mechanism.

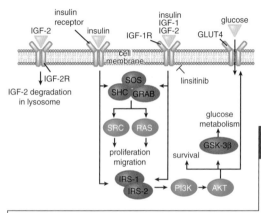

PHYSIOLOGY

- Insulin is a key metabolic regulator and growth factor.
- IGF-*1,2* are structurally similar to insulin.
- IGF-*1R* drives growth.
- IGF-*2R* depletes IGF-2 by endocytosis.

NOTABLE BEHAVIORS IN CANCER

- Hyperinsulinemia due to obesity, diabetes, metabolic syndrome, etc., increases risk of and mortality from cancer
- Glucose transporter (GLUT)4 is overexpressed in pancreatic cancers, possibly linked to castration-resistant phenotype.
- IGF-1R is overexpressed in some cancers, possibly to increase glucose uptake via insulin receptor substrate (IRS)-1-dependent membrane translocation of GLUT.
- IGF levels are prognostic in NSCLC and sarcoma.
- IGF-1R promotes resistance to EGFR drugs by dimerizing with EGFR.
- IGF-1R drugs have limited clinical activity, significant adverse effects, for example, hyperglycemia.

- Insulin-like growth factor family includes two growth factors (IGF-1, IGF-2) and two receptors (IGF-1R, IGF-2R).
- IGF-1 and IGF-2 are polypeptide hormones structurally similar to insulin. IGF-IR, IGF-2R, and insulin receptors are also structurally similar and are able to form heterodimers.
- IGF-1R is activated by IGF-1, IGF-2, and insulin and has a strong growth-promoting effect.
- IGF-2R does not trigger signaling, but regulates extracellular IRS-2 levels through receptor-mediated endocytosis and degradation. Upon phosphorylation, IGF-1R recruits and phosphorylates adaptor proteins IRS-1, IRS-2, and SRC homology 2 domain-containing protein (SHC).
- IRS-1 acts as a second messenger within cell to stimulate transcription of insulin-related genes (e.g., ELK1, glycogen synthase-3 [GSK3]) via PI3K and RAS pathways and also initiates the translocation of GLUT to the cell surface where it facilitates transport of glucose into the cell.
- IRS-2 plays a critical role in cellular motility response, and SHC stimulates activation of MAPK pathway.
- Compared with normal cells, cancer cells have an increased need for glucose, which alters cellular metabolism (i.e., Warburg effect).

- Increased levels of IGF-1R are expressed in certain types of cancer cells (e.g., prostate, pancreatic), which can lead to increased uptake of glucose from blood into tumor. However, IGF-1R expression does not consistently correlate with disease control in heterogeneous groups of patients treated with anti-IGF-1R monoclonal antibodies (mAbs).
- IGF ligand (IGF-1) levels have been shown to have predictive value in NSCLC and sarcoma, but correlation between ligand level and tumor microenvironment has not been established.
- In the presence of epidermal growth factor (EGF) inhibitors, IGF-1R can dimerize with EGFR, allowing pathway signaling to resume, leading to resistance of these inhibitors.
- Although there is compelling preclinical evidence, only limited clinical activity of IGF-1R inhibition has been observed in several tumor types, including NSCLC and breast cancer. More favorable outcomes were observed in patients with sarcoma.
- Furthermore, common adverse effects of IGF-1R inhibition that include hyperglycemia (pituitary feedback loop), nausea, vomiting, fatigue, anorexia, and skin reactions have limited the U.S. Food and Drug Administration (FDA) approval of any IGF-1R pathway inhibitors so far.

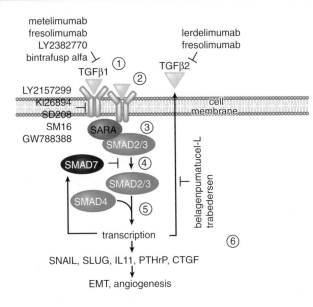

CLASSICAL SIGNALING

1. Activation of transforming growth factor-beta (TGFβ) receptors
2. Oligomerization
3. Phosphorylation of SMAD2/3
4. Translocation of SMADs to nucleus
5. Expression of target genes, for example, cyclin-dependent kinase (CDK) inhibitors
6. Physiologic response, for example, cytoskeletal rearrangement, remodeling of extracellular matrix

NOTABLE BEHAVIORS IN CANCER

- TGFβ is upregulated in some cancers with programmed cell death ligand 1 (PD-L1), inhibits anticancer immunity, and contributes to poor prognosis.
- SMAD4 deletion is common in pancreatic cancers, inactivating mutations in liver, colorectal cancer.
- Germline SMAD4 lesion is linked to hereditary juvenile polyposis.
- TGFβ induces tumor cell migration and boosts epithelial to mesenchymal transition.
- TGFβ is a powerful suppressor of innate and adaptive immunity, promoting immune surveillance by tumor cells.

- TGFβ signaling pathway plays a critical role in cell growth, differentiation, and development. TGFβ stimulates proliferation of mesenchymal cells, but inhibits proliferation of epithelial cells.
- In cancer, TGFβ inhibits immune response against cancer, while stimulating stromal cells to proliferate.
- Signaling is initiated by interaction of the ligand with the receptor and oligomerization of serine/threonine TGFβ receptor kinases and phosphorylation of the cytoplasmic signaling molecules SMAD2 and SMAD3.
- SMAD transcription factors are phosphorylated and translocated to nucleus where they stimulate expression of genes encoding CDK inhibitors or proteins involved in the formation and remodeling of extracellular matrix.
- Activation of pathway is counteracted by inhibitory SMADs (e.g., SMAD7), which are encoded by gene induced by pathway stimulation (feedback mechanism).
- TGFβ/activin and bone morphogenetic protein (BMP) pathways are modulated by MAPK signaling at a number of levels. Moreover, in certain contexts, TGFβ signaling can also affect

SMAD-independent pathways, including ERK, stress-activated protein kinase/c-Jun NH2-terminal kinase (SAPK/JNK), and p38 MAPK pathways.

- Rho GTPase (RhoA) activates downstream target proteins to prompt rearrangement of the cytoskeletal elements associated with cell growth, migration, and invasion.
- A germline mutation in SMAD4 is known to be associated with hereditary juvenile polyposis syndrome.
- Targeting TGFβ can be done by different drugs that include antisense oligonucleotides (AONs), neutralizing antibodies that inhibit ligand–receptor interactions, receptor domain–immunoglobulin fusions that sequester ligands and prevent binding to receptors, and receptor kinase inhibitors.
  - AONs (target TGFβ2): trabedersen (AP12009) and antisense gene-modified allogenic tumor vaccine: Belagenpumatucel-L (Lucanix) are currently in clinical trials.
  - Antibodies: Fresolimumab (GC-1008)—binds TGFβ1 and TGFβ2; IMC-TR1—targets TβRII
  - TGFβ kinase inhibitors/small-molecule inhibitors: LY2157299 (galunisertib); TEW-7197
- Although TGFβ targeting agents, such as galunisertib, have shown dramatic therapeutic effects in animal cancer models and in some cancer patients, it is still not clear how the therapeutic effect in cancer patients is achieved; currently, there is no predictive biomarker for response to drugs targeting the TGFβ pathway.
- TGFβ and PD-L1 are both upregulated in certain types of cancers, and their overexpression is associated with increased evasion of immune surveillance and contributes to poor prognosis.
- Bintrafusp alfa, a bifunctional fusion protein composed of avelumab, an anti-PD-L1 human mAb, bound to the soluble extracellular domain of TGFβRII, has shown to increase natural killer (NK) cell and cytotoxic T-lymphocyte (CTL) activities inhibiting tumor cell proliferation; it is currently being tested in clinical trials.

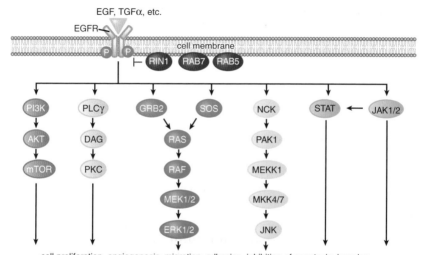

cell proliferation, angiogenesis, migration, adhesion, inhibition of apoptosis, invasion

PHYSIOLOGY
- **Family consists of EGFR (ERBB1), HER2 (ERBB2), HER3 (ERBB3), HER4 (ERBB4).**
- **EGFR, HER2, HER4 are active kinases.**

EGF FAMILY OF RECEPTORS

- The EGF family of receptors are transmembrane RTKs that are frequently overexpressed or mutated in a wide variety of epithelial tumors.
- The EGF or ERBB family consists of EGFR (ERBB1), HER2 (ERBB2), HER3 (ERBB3), and HER4 (ERBB4).
- They are characterized by an extracellular ligand-binding domain and an intracellular tyrosine kinase domain except ERBB3, which has a kinase-deficient intracellular domain.

ACTIVATION OF THE RECEPTORS

- The EGF family of receptors is activated by binding to a ligand resulting in homo- or heterodimerization of the receptors and phosphorylation of the receptors at the cytosolic kinase domain. This results in the recruitment of adapter molecules, leading to activation of signaling pathway cascades downstream.
- One of the well-studied pathways acts through the RAS → rapidly accelerated fibrosarcoma (RAF) → ERK cascade. The other major pathway involves the lipid kinase PI3K, AKT, and mammalian target of rapamycin (mTOR). The activation of these pathways leads to cell growth, proliferation, differentiation, and migration.
- The receptor is trafficked through the early and late endosomes and lysosomes, where it is degraded by proteases. This regulation mechanism driven by RAB5, RIN1, and RAB7 ensures downregulation of receptor signaling when not required.

LIGANDS

- EGFR (ERBB1) has seven known ligands: EGF, TGFα, heparin-binding EGF-like growth factor (HBEGF), amphiregulin (AREG), β-cellulin (BTC), epiregulin (EREG), and epigen (EPGN). EGF and TGFα are the most common and most characterized.

- Interestingly, ERBB2 (HER2) does not have a ligand. ERBB2 can heterodimerize with EGFR, ERBB3, and ERBB4, functioning through activation of other receptor family members.
- Neuregulin 1 and 2 bind ERBB3 to activate it, whereas EGF, BTC, and neuregulins (1–4) bind ERBB4.

EGFR SIGNALING IN CANCER

- Dysregulation of EGFR signaling is seen in cancer.
- EGFR kinase domain mutations are commonly seen in lung cancer. These result in constitutive activation of the EGF receptor.
- EGFR overexpression is commonly seen in head and neck squamous cell carcinoma (80%–90%), NSCLC (~60%), triple-negative breast cancer (~60%), colon cancer (>90%), and glioblastoma (~50%). EGFR overexpression can occur by increase in copy number or increase in protein expression.
- Other mechanisms of signaling dysregulation include defective downregulation of the receptor (caused by CBL mutations and seen in EGFRvIII) and cross-talk with other receptors (such as other ERBB family members and G-protein-coupled receptors or GPCRs).

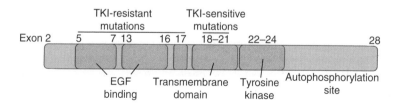

Notable behaviors in cancer	• Overexpressed in head and neck squamous cell carcinoma (80%–90%), NSCLC (~60%), triple-negative breast cancer (~60%), colon cancer (>90%), and glioblastoma (~50%). • Constitutively active mutants common in lung cancer • Normal switch-off mechanisms may be lost • May cross-talk with other receptors	
EGFR-activating mutations	• L858R on exon 21 • in-frame deletion in exon 19	• Account for 90% of activating mutations
	• L861Q (exon 21) • G719X (exon 18) • V765A, T783A (exon 20) • Some in-frame deletion/insertion on exon 20 • T790M: most common lesion that confers resistance to EGFR drugs	
EGFR VIII	• Truncated form after deletion of exons 2–7 by gene rearrangement • Unable to bind ligand, but is constitutively active because of interaction with wild-type EGFR and loss of downregulation mechanism • Preferentially triggers PI3K/AKT, whereas other mutants activate MAPK	

Activating mutations, except exon 20 insertions, hypersensitize cells to EGFR inhibitors. Exon 20 mutations contribute to resistance to EGFR inhibitors.

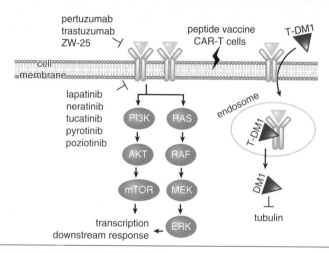

NOTABLE BEHAVIORS IN CANCER

- Overexpression, rather than simple activation, is required for tumorigenic activity.
- Overexpression may alter the repertoire of HER2-containing dimers, resulting in altered signaling.
- Overexpression deregulates cell cycle, polarity, and adhesion.
- Overexpression elicits oncogene addiction, the basis of drug activity.

LESIONS IN CANCER

- Overexpressed/amplified in breast (~30% of tumors), esophageal (~17%), lung (~3%), ovarian (~2%–66%), colorectal (~3%), prostate, salivary gland, bladder cancer
- In-frame A775_G776insYVMA in exon 20 seen in NSCLC
- Activating missense mutations in kinase domain seen in breast, lung, colorectal cancers
- Activating mutations in extracellular domain, for example, S310Y and S310F, are seen in ~1%–2% lung and breast cancers, some colorectal and ovarian cancers.

- HER2 (ERBB2) is the second member of the EGFR family of receptors.
- HER2 heterodimerizes with EGFR as well as ERBB3.
- ERBB2/HER2 is often overexpressed/amplified in various cancer types such as breast (~30% of tumors), esophageal (~17% of tumors), lung (~3%), ovarian (~2%–66%), colorectal cancer (~3%). Amplification is also seen in prostate cancer, salivary gland tumors, and bladder cancers.
- *ERBB2* gene mutations are drivers of several cancer types. In NSCLC, ERBB2 exon 20 in-frame insertion/duplication A775_G776insYVMA is the most prevalent.
- Missense activating mutations in tyrosine kinase domains are seen in breast, lung, and colorectal cancers predominantly.
- Extracellular domain mutations causing enhanced kinase activity such as ERBB2 S310Y and ERBB2 S310F are seen in ~1% to 2% lung and breast cancers, and also a small proportion of colorectal and ovarian cancers.

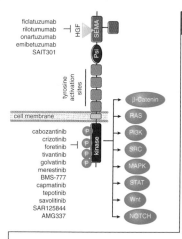

NOTABLE BEHAVIORS IN CANCER

- Deregulation linked to tumor growth, metastasis, poor prognosis
- Hepatocyte growth factor (HGF) lesions linked to kidney, liver, gastric, esophageal, breast, brain, and melanoma
- Cancer stem cells seem to reacquire MET expression, which is normally exclusive to stem and progenitor cells.
- MET activation synergizes with INK4a/ alternate reading frame (ARF) inactivation in rhabdomyosarcoma.
- MET amplification and exon 14 skipping drive NSCLC progression and resistance to EGFR drugs.
- MET amplification linked to aggressive gastric cancer and poor outcome
- Tumor HGF secretion drives MET expression in melanoma.

- Constitutive activation of the HGF promoter is observed in 51% of African-Americans with breast cancer.
- Circulating HGF levels correlated with poorer survival and are potential markers for both presence of cancer and disease stage.

NORMAL BIOLOGY

- c-MET is a proto-oncogene that encodes for hepatocyte growth factor receptor, also known as MET (HGFR), possessing tyrosine kinase activity.
- HGF is the only known ligand of the MET receptor.
- MET induces several biologic responses that collectively give rise to invasive growth.

ROLE IN CANCER

- Abnormal MET activation in cancer correlates with poor prognosis, where uncontrolled MET triggers tumor growth, angiogenesis, and metastasis.
- MET deregulation (MET and HGF amplifications, MET mutations) has been implicated in many types of cancer, including kidney, liver, gastric, esophageal, breast, brain, and melanoma.
- Usually, only stem cells and progenitor cells express MET, which allows for invasive growth; however, cancer stem cells are thought to hijack the ability of normal stem cells to express MET and thus become the cause of cancer persistence and metastasis.
- MET activates multiple signal transduction pathways, including RAS, PI3K, STAT, Wnt, and NOTCH.
- Inactivation of tumor suppressors INK4a/ARF synergizes with MET activation in rhabdomyosarcoma.
- MET expression is driven by HGF secretions in the tumor cell microenvironment in melanoma.
- In NSCLC, c-MET amplification and exon 14 skipping drive progression and resistance to EGFR inhibitors. In gastric cancers, amplification is associated with aggressive disease and poor outcomes.

Physiology	• Receptor for glial cell line–derived neurotropic factors (GDNF) • Activates MAPK and PI3K pathways similar to EGFR.
Notable behaviors in cancer	• Point mutations drive multiple endocrine neoplasia syndromes (MEN2) and familial medullary thyroid cancer. • Fusion with other proteins may cause constitutive activation, potentially via dimerization. • Fusions associated with radiation exposure, seen in NSCLC, Spitz tumors, breast, colon cancers, ~1/3 of papillary thyroid cancers • Fusion partners include KIF5B, CCDC6, GOLGA5, TRIM24, TRIM27, TRIM33, PRKAR1A, MBD1, KTN1, HOOK3, AKAP13, FKBP15, SPECC1L, ERC1, NCOA4, TBL1XR1, RAB6IP2

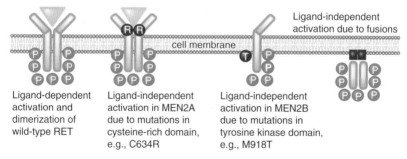

Ligand-dependent activation and dimerization of wild-type RET

Ligand-independent activation in MEN2A due to mutations in cysteine-rich domain, e.g., C634R

Ligand-independent activation in MEN2B due to mutations in tyrosine kinase domain, e.g., M918T

Ligand-independent activation due to fusions

(Adapted from Romei C, Ciampi R, Elisei R. A comprehensive overview of the role of the RET proto-oncogene in thyroid carcinoma. *Nat Rev Endocrinol*. 2016;12(4):192–202.)

- REarranged during Transfection (RET) receptor can activate MAPK and PI3K pathways similar to EGFR.
- RET is a receptor for the GDNF family of extracellular ligands.

ROLE IN CANCER

- Point mutations in RET give rise to MEN2 and familial medullary thyroid cancer.
- Chromosomal rearrangements that create a fusion between RET and other proteins can cause constitutive activation of RET receptor.
- Fusions of RET with other genes have been identified in multiple malignancies.
  - Found in approximately one-third of patients with papillary thyroid cancer. Associated with radiation exposure.
  - RET fusions have also been identified as an oncogenic driver in NSCLC, Spitz tumors, breast, and colon cancers.
  - RET fusion partners include KIF5B, CCDC6, GOLGA5, TRIM24, TRIM27, TRIM33, PRKAR1A, MBD1, KTN1, HOOK3, AKAP13, FKBP15, SPECC1L, ERC1, NCOA4, TBL1XR1, and RAB6IP2. Many of these partners have dimerization motifs, suggesting this as a possible mechanism for RET activation.

Physiology	• Also known as CD246; receptor for insulin • Expressed in brain, testis, small intestine; enhanced expression in developing nervous system; lower expression in adults
Notable behaviors in cancer	• Overactivated following fusion with other genes, typically via constitutive dimerization • Amplification and gene deletions seen in several malignancies, e.g., in 13 of 15 specimens of inflammatory breast cancer • Nonfusion lesions of unknown significance, although mutation and overexpression seen in 40%–100% of neuroblastomas

NOTABLE FUSIONS

Physiology	Partners	Prev. (%)
Lymphoma	NPM, TPM3, TPM4	60
NSCLC	EML4, K1F5B	5
Colorectal	EML4	2
Breast	EML4	2
Renal	EML4, TPM3	2

• NPM binds ss- and dsDNA; drives DNA repair, stabilizes genome
• TPM3 drives muscle contraction
• EML4 modifies microtubules
• K1F5B required to distribute mitochondria, lysosomes

ROLE IN CANCER

- Observed mechanisms of oncogenesis involve overactivation of the ALK receptor through fusion gene formation. The most common is the EML4–ALK fusion, occurring in 2% to 7% of NSCLCs.
- ALK fusions were first discovered in lymphoma. In solid tumors, they are found most commonly in lung adenocarcinoma, but have been identified in Spitz tumors, sarcoma, melanoma, breast, colorectal, esophageal, cholangiocarcinoma, thyroid, neuroblastoma, renal cell, renal medullary, and bladder cancers.
- Fusion partner usually has a domain that induces constitutive dimerization with resultant activation.
- In NSCLC, patients with ALK fusions are usually young with minimal or no smoking history.
- ALK amplifications and gene deletions have been identified in several malignancies. At this time, the significance of nonfusion alterations is unclear.
- Crizotinib was the first-generation ALK inhibitor; second-generation inhibitors include ceritinib, alectinib, and brigatinib; lorlatinib is a third-generation inhibitor.

Physiology	• Regulates cell survival, proliferation, differentiation • Expressed as multiple transcript variants encoding isoforms • Strongly expressed by hematopoietic stem cells, multipotent progenitors, common myeloid progenitors, early thymocyte progenitors; lower levels of expression in common lymphoid progenitors, mast cells, melanocytes, interstitial cells of Cajal in digestive tract
Lesions in Cancer	• Activating mutations linked to GIST, testicular seminoma, mast cell disease, melanoma, acute myeloid leukemia • Primary mutations in exon 11 and 9 linked to sensitivity and intrinsic resistance to imatinib, respectively • Secondary mutations in kinase domain (exons 13–18) linked to acquired resistance to imatinib.

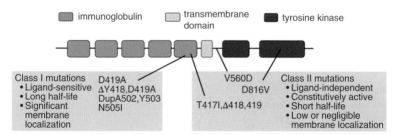

(Adapted from Shi X, Sousa LP, Mandel-Bausch EM, Tome F, Reshetnyak AV, Hadari Y, Schlessinger J, Lax I. Distinct cellular properties of oncogenic KIT receptor tyrosine kinase mutants enable alternative courses of cancer cell inhibition. *Proc Natl Acad Sci U S A.* 2016;113(33):E4784–E4793.)

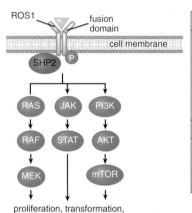

ROS1 — fusion domain

cell membrane

SHP2 — P

RAS → RAF → MEK

JAK → STAT

PI3K → AKT → mTOR

proliferation, transformation, survival

Physiology

- Structurally similar to ALK, but activated by unknown ligand
- Function also unknown, but contains extracellular sequences analogous to cell adhesion proteins, triggers typical RTK pathways
- In normal adults, expression is highest in the kidney, with some expression in stomach, intestines, neural tissue.

Lesions in Cancer

- Fusion with various partners enhances oncogenesis.
- ROS-1 rearrangement relatively rare, seen only in the absence of other known oncogenic driver mutations
- ROS-1 mutation seen in ~2% of NSCLCs

Fusion partners

TPM3	CD74	KDELR2
CEP85L	TFG	ZER
CCDC6	FIG	YWHAE
SLC34A2	SDC4	LRIG3

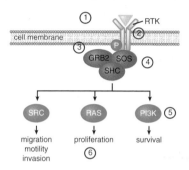

Signaling

1. Activation by growth factors
2. Homo- or heterodimerization
3. Autophosphorylation
4. Recruitment of adaptor proteins
5. Activation of downstream pathways
6. Physiologic response

Oncogenic Mechanisms

- **Activating gain-of-function mutations**
- **Overexpression because of genomic amplification**

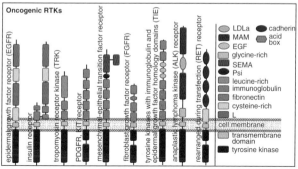

- RTKs are cell surface receptors that function as key regulators of fundamental cellular processes such as proliferation, differentiation, senescence, and migration, among others.
- Binding growth factor ligands to extracellular domain, RTKs induce receptor dimerization (forming either homodimers or heterodimers with other RTKs) followed by their autophosphorylation. This allows for subsequent recruitment of adaptor proteins such as growth factor receptor–bound protein 2 (GRB2), SHC, and Son of Sevenless (SOS) that activate proliferation, survival, and migration pathways (e.g., RAS, PI3K, SRC).
- Tight control of RTK activation is necessary for tissue homeostasis, which is why RTKs constitute one of the biggest classes of oncoproteins.
- Over 20 different classes of RTKs have been identified, including the following that have been previously implicated in cancer initiation and progression: ALK, EGFR, FGFR, IGFR, KIT, MET, PDGFR, RET, TIE, and VEGFR. Each RTK will be discussed in detail in this section.

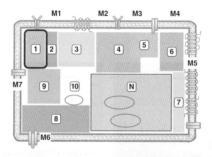

Rapamycin is a naturally occurring "antibiotic" discovered on the Pacific island of Rapa Nui (Easter Island) in the 1970s. This "family" consists of the mTOR complex, PI3K, AKT, phosphatase and tensin homolog (PTEN) and is an important key regulator of the immune system, glucose metabolism, and cell growth.

PI3K activation leads to phosphorylation and activation of AKT, which in turn can activate mTOR. The pathway can be suppressed by tuberous sclerosis (TSC1; hamartin), TSC2 (tuberin), and phosphatidylinositol-3,4,5-trisphosphate 3-phosphatase (PTEN). PI3Ks are divided into three classes according to structural characteristics and substrate specificity. This pathway interacts with IRS to regulate glucose uptake through a series of phosphorylation events. Hyperglycemia and sore mouth are common but manageable side effects in patients taking PI3K inhibitors.

Easter Island is a triangular-shaped Chilean territory in the Pacific Ocean and is known for the remarkable stone head sculptures.

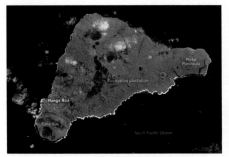

(NASA Earth Observatory image by Jesse Allen, using Landsat data from the U.S. Geological Survey. Available at https://earthobservatory.nasa.gov/images/90027/easter-island)

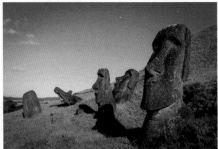

(From Shutterstock.)

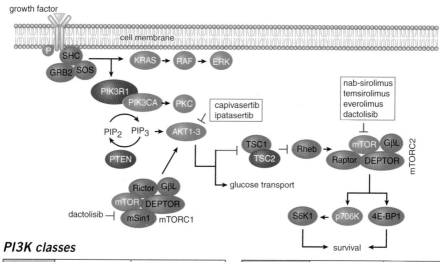

PI3K classes

Class IA	Catalytic	PIK3CA,B,D
	Regulatory	PI3KR1,2,3
Class II	Catalytic	PIK3C2A,2B,2G

Class IB	Catalytic	PIK3CG
	Regulatory	PI3KR5
Class III	Catalytic	PIK3C3

- PI3K/protein kinase B (PKB or AKT)/mTOR pathway is a key regulator of normal cellular processes. Aberrant activation of this pathway leads to survival and proliferation of tumor cells.
- PI3K activation leads to phosphorylation and activation of AKT, which in turn can activate mTOR. The pathway can be suppressed by TSC1 (hamartin), TSC2 (tuberin), and PTEN.
- PI3Ks are divided into three classes according to structural characteristics and substrate specificity:
  - Class I
    - Class IA PI3Ks: heterodimers consisting of a p110 catalytic subunit (isoforms p110α, p110β, and p110δ encoded by the genes *PIK3CA*, *PIK3CB*, and *PIK3CD*, respectively) and a p85 regulatory subunit (isoforms p85α [and slice variants p55α and p50α] encoded by PIK3R1, p85β encoded by PIK3R2, and p85γ encoded by PIK3R3)
    - Class IB PI3Ks: heterodimers consisting of a p110γ (encoded by PIK3CG) and a p101 regulatory subunit (encoded by PIK3R5)
  - Class II: monomers with a single catalytic subunit (isoforms PI3KC2α, PI3KC2β, and PI3KC2γ encoded by PIK3C2A, PIK3C2B, and PIK3C2G, respectively)
  - Class III: single catalytic subunit VPS34 (encoded by *PIK3C3* gene)
- This pathway interacts with the IRS to regulate glucose uptake through a series of phosphorylation events. A common side effect in patients taking PI3Ks inhibitors is hyperglycemia.

Molecule	Notable Behaviors in Cancer
PIK3CA	Activating missense mutations occur throughout, with most in hotspots, e.g., E542K, E545K in exon 9; H1047R in exon 20
PIK3R1	• Substitutions, in-frame insertions, deletions in iSH2 domain that impair inhibitory activity against catalytic subunit • Somatic mutations prevalent in endometrial, glioma, colon cancer • Suppressed in some cancers
PIK3CB	Seen in breast and castration-resistant prostate cancer
PIK3CD PIK3CG	Typically not mutated, but amplified or overexpressed
PIK3R2	• Somatic mutations in endometrial, colorectal cancer, but no hotspot • Overexpression in breast, colon cancer
PIK3C2B	• Like PIK3C2A, expressed in tumor cells • Mutations seen in NSCLC • Amplification in glioblastoma
AKT1	• E17K in melanoma, breast, colorectal, endometrial, ovarian, squamous cell lung cancer; amplification in gastric cancer
AKT2	• Mutations in colorectal cancer; amplification in head and neck, pancreatic, ovarian, breast cancers
AKT3	• Amplification in melanoma, breast, endometrial, ovarian cancer
PTEN	• Germline mutations linked to inherited PTEN hamartoma tumor syndrome (PHTS) that increase the risk of breast, thyroid, endometrial cancer
TSC1/2	• Mutations linked to bladder, kidney cancers

TARGETING AKT MUTATIONS

- AKT (also known as PKB) is a serine–threonine protein kinase expressed as three isoforms AKT1, AKT2, and AKT3 (encoded by the genes *PKBα*, *PKBβ*, and *PKBγ*, respectively).
- Activation through mutation has been reported for all three isoforms (AKT1, AKT2, AKT3) and activation through amplification has been reported for two isoforms only (AKT1, AKT2). They affect survival, proliferation, and apoptosis of cancer cells with additional effects on tumor-induced angiogenesis through activation of other kinases (e.g., BCL-2-associated death promoter [BAD], mouse double minute 2 [MDM2], GSK3β).
  - AKT1 is involved in cell survival and growth.
    - Mutation E17K in AKT1 has been identified in melanoma, breast, colorectal, endometrial, and ovarian cancers.
    - Mutation is most common in breast, colorectal, and squamous cell lung carcinoma cancers; amplification is most common in gastric cancer.
  - AKT2 is involved in invasiveness and insulin responsiveness.
    - Mutation is most common in colorectal cancer; amplification is common in head and neck, pancreatic, ovary, and breast cancers.
  - AKT3 is involved in survival and apoptosis.
    - Amplification is common in a wide variety of cancers, for example, breast, endometrial, ovarian, and melanoma.

TARGETING PTEN AND TSC ALTERATIONS

- PTEN is a lipid phosphatase that removes phosphate on the three positions of PIP3 and converts it back to PIP2.
- Germline mutations in the *PTEN* gene are associated with inherited cancer predisposition syndromes collectively known as PHTS (e.g., Cowden syndrome and Bannayan–Riley–Ruvalcaba syndrome); individuals with PHTS have an increased incidence of breast, thyroid, and endometrial cancers.
- Preclinical data suggest mTOR inhibitors exhibit activity against PTEN alterations.
- TSC1 or hamartin and TSC2 or tuberin proteins are tumor suppressors in the PI3K pathway.
- TSC1–TSC2 (hamartin–tuberin) complex is a critical negative regulator of mTORC1 through its GAP (GTPase-activating protein) activity toward the small G-protein Rheb (Ras homolog enriched in brain).
- Germline TSC1/2 mutations have been linked to bladder and kidney cancers.
- Loss of TSC1/2 function leads to overactivity of mTOR; therefore, mTOR inhibitors may show activity against TSC alterations.

PHYSIOLOGY

- Considered to be class IV PI3Ks
- Activated in response to growth factors and nutrients
- A master regulator of metabolic homeostasis, protein and lipid synthesis, glycolysis, mitochondria biogenesis, lysosome biogenesis, proteasome assembly, and autophagy

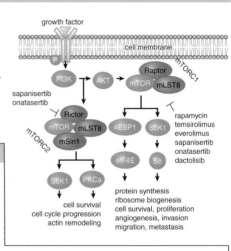

NOTABLE BEHAVIORS IN CANCER

- Mutations (potentially hyperactivating, usually rapamycin-sensitive) detected in colorectal, endometrial, lung cancers
- Amplification of other subunits, for example, raptor, has been seen.
- Also activated by oncogenic activation of upstream regulators, for example, RTKs, PI3K
- Mediates metabolic reprogramming to ensure tumor cell survival and proliferation; also responds to upstream metabolic changes, for example, increased glucose or amino acid uptake
- mTORC inhibitors are being tested in combination with other drugs that interfere with cellular metabolism, for example, the diabetes drug metformin.

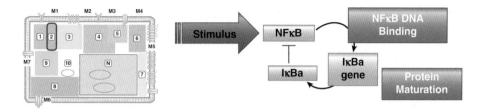

Nuclear factor kappa B (NF-κB) is an ancient protein transcription factor and considered a regulator of innate immunity. The NF-κB signaling pathway links pathogenic signals and cellular danger signals, thus organizing cellular resistance to invading pathogens.

NF-κB is a network hub responsible for complex biologic signaling and is considered a master regulator of evolutionarily conserved biochemical cascades. Other factors are also translocated into the mitochondria and are involved in modulating expression.

NF-κB Pathway

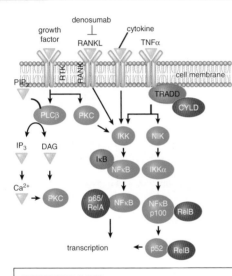

NOTABLE BEHAVIORS IN CANCER

- Osteoclasts, which express RANK, are aberrantly activated in metastatic bone cancer.
- NF-κB links chronic inflammation to cancer.
- NF-κB lesions are typical in lymphoid cancers, rarer in solid cancers.
- NF-κB may be constitutively activated by lesions in upstream regulators or by deregulated secretion of cytokines and other stimuli.
- Constitutive NF-κB activation elicits chemo- and radio-resistance.
- Depending on context, NF-κB can trigger or suppress tumorigenesis.

PHYSIOLOGY

- Cytokine receptors triggered by interferons (e.g., IFNα,β,γ); interleukins (e.g., IL-2)
- RANKL expressed on stromal cells, osteoblasts, T cells
- RANK expressed on osteoclasts, dendritic cells; regulates immune signaling

G-Protein-Coupled Receptors

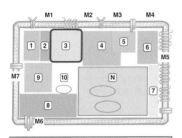

Nobel Prizes in 1994 and 2012

GPCRs are "seven-transmembrane" globular proteins that make up the largest and most diverse group of cell surface receptors. They are named for their binding to guanosine diphosphate (GDP). The conversion of GDP to the triphosphate GTP is the "on/off" switch that positively ($+$) or negatively ($-$) affects hundreds of "druggable" enzyme cascades.

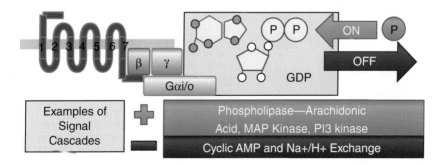

Examples of Signal Cascades

$+$ Phospholipase—Arachidonic Acid, MAP Kinase, PI3 kinase

$-$ Cyclic AMP and Na+/H+ Exchange

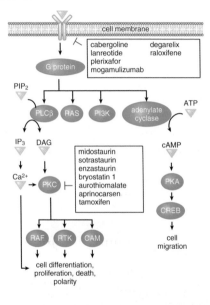

PHYSIOLOGY

- Large family of receptors that regulate multiple signaling pathways
- Activated by diverse ligands, for example, chemokines, hormones, neurotransmitters
- Targeted by the most successful drugs to manage pain, inflammation, neurologic, and metabolic disorders

NOTABLE BEHAVIORS IN CANCER

- Downstream effector PKC frequently dysregulated in cancers
- Deregulated levels of GPCR ligands in the circulation or tumor environment trigger sustained activation, driving tumor growth
- GPCR mutations seen in ~20% of cancers; constitutively active G-protein mutants may drive carcinogenesis.

EMERGING TARGETS OF ANTICANCER DRUGS

- Chemokine, lysophospholipid receptors
- Protease-activated, E-prostanoid receptors
- Smoothened (SMO), Frizzled (FZD) receptors
- GPCRs that regulate Hippo, "transactivate" RTKs

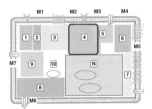

Since the 1980s, the MAP kinases have been an important source of cell signal research. They are specific to the amino acids serine and threonine and control responses to cellular stress: mitogens, heat shock, and inflammatory cytokines. MAPK/ERK regulates cell proliferation, differentiation, mitosis, and apoptosis.

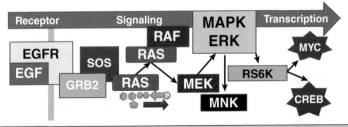

The MAPK "Cascade": Epidermal Growth Factor Receptor (**EGFR**); Growth factor receptor–bound protein 2 (**GRB2**); Son of Sevenless (**SOS**); RAS (**RA**t **S**arcoma virus), a small GTPase that is related to G proteins. **R**apidly **A**ccelerated **F**ibrosarcoma (**RAF**); **MEK is the MAP Kinase Kinase that activates MAPK/ERK. MNKs are downstream effector kinases; RS6K** is Ribosomal **S6** Kinase; **MYK is named for** **MY**elo**C**ytomatosis **avian** virus. **CREB is Cyclic AMP Response Element–Binding Protein.**

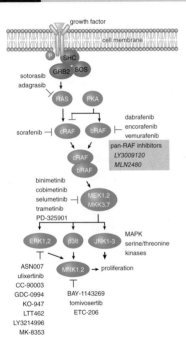

NOTABLE BEHAVIORS IN CANCER

- Sustained pathway signaling following oncogenic activation
- RAS mutations present in up to 30% of cancers
- Constitutively active KRAS (mutated in codons 12, 13, and 61) frequent in pancreatic, colon, lung cancer; KRAS mutations most common Ras lesions (25%–30%)
- HRAS mutations most frequent in bladder cancer, seminoma, Hurthle cell carcinoma
- NRAS mutations common in leukemia, melanoma, thyroid, rectal, follicular cancers
- CRAF overexpressed in lung, liver, prostate, neuroendocrine, myeloid leukemia
- BRAF seen in melanoma (30%–60%), thyroid cancer (30%–50%), colorectal cancer (5%–20%), of which 905 is V600E.
- MEK1/2 mutation and BRAF amplification in V600E cancers may confer resistance to MEK drugs.

- Signaling through the RAS/RAF/MEK/ERK (MAPK) pathway is essential for the proliferation of normal cells as well as for many cancer cells.
- Activation of pathway occurs through growth factor binding to RTKs and also by other extra- and intracellular stimuli.
- MAPK are involved in directing cellular responses to a variety of stimuli and help regulate proliferation, gene expression, and apoptosis, among others.
- In cancer cells, pathway signaling is often heightened as a consequence of oncogenic activation of RTKs, RAS, or RAF. The pathway cascade ultimately leads to ERK activation.
- MAPK kinases activated by MEK1/2 were previously known as ERK1 and ERK2 (extracellular signal–regulated kinases). MAPKs are serine/threonine kinases that include ERK1/2, P38 kinase, ERK5, and c-Jun (JNK1/2/3) kinases.

TARGETING BRAF
- RAF kinase family is serine/threonine-specific protein kinases that mediate signal transduction in MAPK pathway. Raf kinase family consists of three isoforms: RAF-1/CRAF, BRAF, ARAF.
- All Raf proteins share MEK1/2 kinases as a substrate.
- CRAF overexpression is found in a variety of primary human cancers: lung, liver, prostate, neuroendocrine tumors, and myeloid leukemia.
- BRAF mutations are found in melanoma (30%–60%), thyroid cancer (30%–50%), colorectal cancer (5%–20%).
- The most common BRAF mutation, valine (V) is substituted for by glutamate (E) at codon 600 (now referred to as V600E) in the activation segment, which accounts for 90% of BRAF mutations that are seen in human cancers. BRAF V600E mutation indicates poor prognosis in colorectal cancers.

TARGETING KRAS
- Specific KRASG12C inhibitors are now approved or in clinical trials, e.g., sotorasib and adagrasib.
- KRASG12D or pan-RAS inhibitors are upcoming.

TARGETING MEK
- MAP kinase kinases or MAPKK (also known as MEK or MAP2K) is a family of kinase enzymes in the RAS MAPK pathway.
- Inhibitors of MEK1/2 have shown efficacy in BRAF- and KRAS-mutated cancers.
- Mutations in MEK1/2 and BRAF amplification have been identified as potential mechanisms of resistance to MEK inhibitors in cancer cells harboring BRAF V600E mutation.

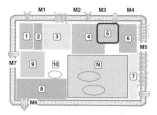

Peyton Rous discovered Rous sarcoma virus (RSV) in the early 1900s working with naturally occurring tumors in chickens. He found that by injecting RSV as a cell filtrate, RSV could induce solid tumors in closely related healthy fowl. He was awarded the Nobel Prize in 1966 for the discovery that viruses could cause tumors and cancer.

The genetic material of RSV—RSV is derived from the more common avian leukosis virus (ALV)—is ribonucleic acid (RNA), which can be transcribed into DNA by reverse transcriptase. Once incorporated into host DNA, proto-oncogene cellular c-Src function increases. Src is a nine-member family of nonreceptor tyrosine kinases. Src triggers downstream phosphorylation signaling and is linked to cancer promotion and carcinogenesis. Bishop and Varmus were awarded the Nobel Prize in 1989 for their work that included the startling discovery that one Src gene is normally present in virtually all animals and is "hijacked" as part of the process of carcinogenesis.

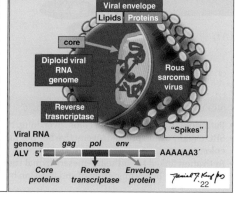

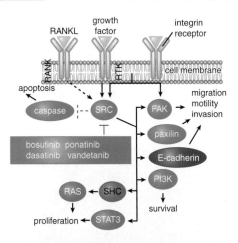

PHYSIOLOGY
- SRC is a nonreceptor tyrosine kinase that triggers phosphorylation cascades.
- Integrins mediate cell–matrix interactions, attachment of actin cytoskeleton at focal adhesion sites.
- May trigger or protect cells from apoptosis
- SRC may also act as direct effector of G proteins, and thus of GPCRs.

NOTABLE BEHAVIORS IN CANCER

- Pathway activated in ~50% of colon, liver, lung, breast, pancreatic tumors
- SRC usually overexpressed/overactive but not mutated, although mutations have been seen in colon cancer
- Activation linked to epithelial–mesenchymal transition, malignant transformation, and, subsequently, heavy migration of and invasion by cancer cells

- E-cadherin mutations seen in gastric, prostate cancers
- Altered integrin expression enables metastasis.
- SRC may also control tumor angiogenesis.
- SRC (short for sarcoma) is a family of nonreceptor protein tyrosine kinases that play an important role in the regulation of cell adhesion, invasion, and motility by phosphorylating specific tyrosine residues in other proteins such as RAS, CAMs (e.g., FAK, focal adhesion protein), and cadherins (e.g., E-cadherins).
- FAK activation by SRC is particularly important for cell adhesion and motility that leads to metastasis.
- SRC activates RAS pathway via SHC.
- SRC also activates E-cadherin, a tumor suppressor that regulates cell invasion.
- Activation of pathway is observed in approximately 50% tumors from colon, liver, lung, breast, and pancreas.
- SRC kinases are usually overexpressed or overactive in cancers, but not mutated, although mutations have been identified (e.g., colon cancer).
  - Activation is often associated with advanced stages of cancer, where cells become highly invasive and migratory.
  - Mutations in E-cadherin have been identified in gastric and prostate cancers.
- SRC is activated by RTK, integrin, VEGFR, and RANK/tumor necrosis factor (TNF)-11.
- Integrin receptors are a family of more than 24 heterodimers that mediate interactions between extracellular matrix and cells and also intracellular signal transduction.
- Altered integrin receptor expression in cancer cells can enable the mobility of metastasizing cells.
- Integrins mediate cell–matrix interactions by binding to extracellular matrix.
- Provide a focus to organize attachment of actin cytoskeleton at focal adhesion contacts

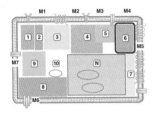

Rolf Kemler et al. (late 1980s) isolated β-catenin and two other molecules, associated with cell adhesion (E-cadherin).

Wnt (**W**ingless fruit fly **Int**egrated) proteins bind to FZD membrane seven-pass receptors. β-Catenin (Axin, Dsh, APC, GSK3, casein kinase-1 [CK1]) is phosphorylated and targeted in the "off state" and for degradation. FZD inhibits phosphorylation and β-catenin accumulates in the nucleus, binds to T-cell factors (TCF), and regulates the cell cycle.

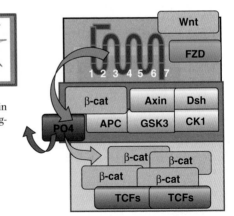

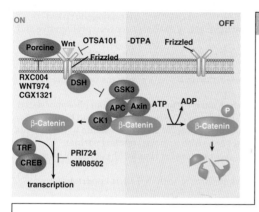

PHYSIOLOGY

- Pivotal in cell proliferation, differentiation, growth, survival, development, regeneration, homeostasis
- Regulates stemness, including of cancer stem cells; can induce dedifferentiation of intestinal epithelial cells into stem cells
- Controls proliferation, maturation, and differentiation of T cells and dendritic cells
- Deregulation drives cancer, metabolic disorders, degenerative diseases

- β-Catenin overexpression, impaired β-catenin degradation, overexpression of Wnt ligands seen in cancer cells
- Persistent signaling because of loss of APC is a key driver of colorectal cancer.
- Wnt signaling activated in 50% of breast cancers and linked to poorer overall survival

- Wnt signaling delays senescence because of BRAFV^{600E} or NRAS^{Q61K}, increasing the risk of developing melanoma; mediates phenotypic switching in melanomas between proliferative and invasive states.
- The Wnt signaling pathway is pivotal in cell proliferation, differentiation, growth, survival, development, regeneration, and homeostasis.
- Signaling is initiated by binding of the Wnt proteins to their seven-pass transmembrane receptors called FZD, which then activates β-catenin.
- In the absence of the ligand, the Wnt pathway is in an "off" state with β-catenin phosphorylated and targeted for degradation. In the "on" state, however, FZD is activated by ligand binding, which then inhibits phosphorylation and results in the translocation of β-catenin to the nucleus.
- β-Catenin initiates the transcription of its target gene with a nuclear binding partner, transcription factors of the TCF/lymphoid enhancer factor (Lef) family. These regulate the cell cycle including c-myc and CCND1.
- Porcupine protein (PORCN), located in the endoplasmic reticulum (ER), is important for processing Wnt ligand secretion.
- Deregulation of Wnt signaling contributes to the disease states such as cancer, metabolic diseases, and also degenerative diseases. Thus, inhibitors of this pathway could be used to reverse the pathologic state.
- Dysregulation of the pathway in cancer cells may be associated with mutations in β-catenin that result in overexpression, deficiencies in β-catenin destruction complex, and overexpression of Wnt ligands.
- Small-molecule inhibitors have been used to target the Wnt signaling pathway by targeting cytoplasmic proteins, transcription factors, and/or other coactivators.

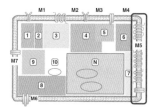

In 1933, Thomas Morgan Hunt received the Nobel Prize for research on *Drosophila melanogaster*—fruit fly genes (FFG). Many of these genes are also fundamental to normal human development because they are mutated and "hijacked" in the process of carcinogenesis. Mutated FFGs are important new drug targets.

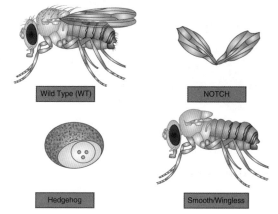

Wild Type (WT)

NOTCH

Hedgehog

Smooth/Wingless

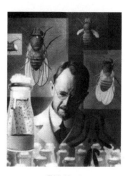

T.M. Hunt

(Courtesy of the Caltech Archives.)

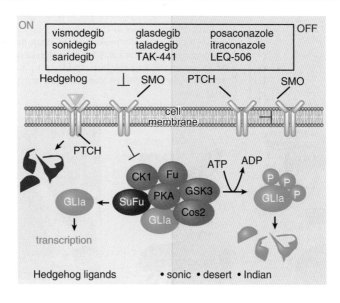

PHYSIOLOGY
- Canonical hedgehog (Hh) signaling occurs mostly in primary cilia (PC), which are immotile but are sensors for mechanical forces, chemicals, light, osmolarity, temperature, gravity.
- Inactive or poorly active in adults except during wound healing, other tissue repair
- Mediates progenitor/stem cell renewal
- Inappropriately activated in basal cell, brain, gastrointestinal, lung, breast, prostate cancer, one-third of malignant tumors
- Activation boosts antiapoptotic genes, angiogenic factors (angiopoietin-1,2), metastatic genes, cyclins D1,B1
- Suppresses apoptotic, cell adhesion, tight junction molecules
- Aberrant activation because of mutations in pathway components or sustained autocrine, paracrine activation
- Paracrine Hh signaling promotes tumorigenesis.
- Sensitive to environmental toxins, for example, piperonyl butoxide, which is common in household and agricultural pesticides

- The Hh pathway can be simplified into four fundamental components: (a) the ligand Hh, (b) the receptor Patched (Patch), (c) the signal transducer Smo, and (d) the effector transcription factor (Gli).
- Canonical Hh signaling occurs predominantly in the PC (Ng and Curran, 2011). PC are tubulin-polymerized immotile cilia that assemble from the centriole at the end of mitosis.
- Components of the Hh pathway concentrate in PC (Ramsbottom and Pownall, 2016; Roy, 2012), and a complex PC trafficking system regulates the interaction of Hh pathway components to enhance, or block, the Hh-initiated signal.

- **OFF State:** In the absence of Hh ligand, the receptor Patch prevents a GPCR-like protein—Smo—from entering the PC, repressing Smo activity.
- This allows the sequential phosphorylation of Gli by several kinases: protein kinase A (PKA), GSK3β, and CK1.
- Phosphorylated Gli is susceptible for ubiquitination by Skp-Cullin-F-box (SCF) protein/β-transducin repeat–containing protein (TrCP), which primes Gli to limited degradation in the proteasome.
- **ON State:** When Hh binds to Patch, it removes Patch from the PC, allowing Smo to enter the PC. The complex Hh–Patch is degraded in vesicles in the cytoplasm. The entry of Smo into the PC allows Smo activation.
- Active Smo abrogates phosphorylation and subsequent degradation of Gli. Full-length Gli translocates to the nucleus where it acts as a transcription factor for several target genes.
- Of note, Shh, Ihh, and Dhh ligands similarly activate the Hh pathway. Gli-1 does not undergo proteasomal degradation, and in the absence of ligand, Gli-2 is preferentially completely degraded in the proteasome, whereas Gli-3 is partially degraded, and hence Gli-1 and Gli-2 act mostly as transcription promoters and Gli-3 can act as a transcription repressor.
- Many human cancers, including brain, gastrointestinal, lung, breast, and prostate cancers, demonstrate inappropriate activation of this pathway.
- Paracrine Hh signaling from the tumor to the surrounding stroma has been shown to promote tumorigenesis.
- Targeted inhibition of Hh signaling may prove effective in the treatment and prevention of many types of human cancers.

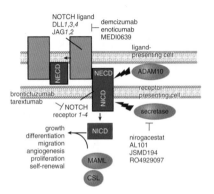

PHYSIOLOGY

- Essential for the development of nervous, cardiovascular, endocrine, respiratory system
- Signaling can be modified by glycosylation and fucosylation of NOTCH receptors, which can affect ligand–receptor interactions.
- Signaling also depends on endocytosis and trafficking of ligands and receptors, which can determine concentrations at cell surface.

CANCER-LINKED LESIONS IN NOTCH RECEPTORS

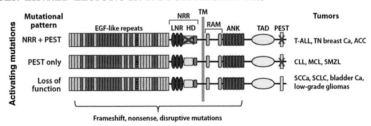

(Republished with permission of Annual Reviews, Inc., from Aster JC, Pear WS, Blacklow SC. The varied roles of Notch in cancer. *Annu Rev Pathol.* 2017 Jan 24;12:245-275.)

- NOTCH is a family of four transmembrane receptors (NOTCH 1–4) that are involved in cell–cell interaction and is found in most multicellular organisms.
- NOTCH signaling is critical to the differentiation and maintenance of several organs that include skin, blood, intestine, liver, and muscle.
- In cancers, mutations in NOTCH can be either activating or inactivating, resulting in oncogenic activity or loss of tumor suppressive function, respectively.
- The NOTCH receptor can be broadly structured into four regions: extracellular domain (NECD), transmembrane domain, intracellular domain (NICD), and the PEST domain located at the C-terminus.
- Two types of NOTCH ligands are known: Delta-like ligands (DLL1, DLL3, DLL4) and Jagged-like ligands (JAG1 and JAG2).
- The binding of the NOTCH ligand to its receptor results in a sequence of two proteolytic events. First, an ADAM family metalloprotease called ADAM10 cleaves the NOTCH protein just outside the plasma membrane. This releases the NECD that will continue to interact with the ligand.
- After the first cleavage, an enzyme called γ-secretase cleaves the remaining part of the NOTCH protein, releasing the NICD from the plasma membrane that translocates to the nucleus.
- In the nucleus, it interacts with DNA where it binds with transcription factors (RBP-J/CSL) and coactivators (Mastermind family, MamL) to induce transcription of target genes, promoting cell proliferation, differentiation, growth, migration, angiogenesis, and self-renewal.

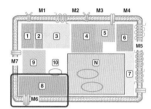

Caspases are activated by DRs and cellular "stress." They work through a network of intermediate molecules to cause cell death: Bid, BCL-2/BCL-Xl, ICAD, IAPS, Smac/Diablo, Omi/HtrA2, cytochrome c, Apaf1, AIF.

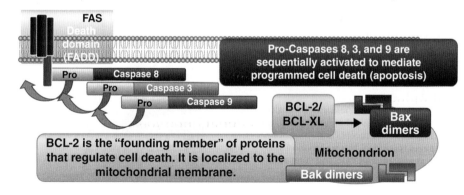

FAS

Death domain (FADD)

Pro | Caspase 8

Pro | Caspase 3

Pro | Caspase 9

Pro-Caspases 8, 3, and 9 are sequentially activated to mediate programmed cell death (apoptosis)

BCL-2/ BCL-XL → **Bax dimers**

BCL-2 is the "founding member" of proteins that regulate cell death. It is localized to the mitochondrial membrane.

Mitochondrion

Bak dimers

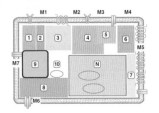

> JAK-STAT inhibitors are used in the treatment of autoimmune diseases (rheumatoid arthritis and ulcerative colitis) as well as myeloproliferative disorders (polycythemia vera/essential thrombocytosis).

JAK/STAT has three main components:

1. Receptor is activated by cytokines or other chemical messengers.
2. JAKs (named because of its two nearly identical sequences) attached to the receptor bind phosphates and attract STAT proteins.
3. STATs form dimers and then translocate into nucleus where they bind to promoters, enhancers, and epigenetic regions to control transcription of target genes, microRNAs, and long noncoding RNAs.

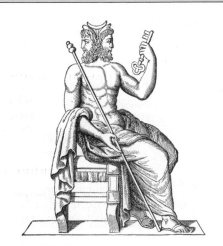

(From Alamy.)

- Among STAT target genes are those encoding SOCS (suppressor of cytokine signaling) factors, which inhibit JAK and contribute to termination of STAT signals.
- STATs can also induce apoptosis mainly by transcriptional activation of genes that encode proteins that trigger cell death process such as BCL-XL (B-cell lymphoma extra-large) and caspases (cysteine-dependent aspartate-directed proteases).
- Signaling through STAT factors in cancers can vary widely because of the many different STATs (e.g., STAT5 in hematologic cancers; STAT3 in breast cancer, head and neck cancer).
- STAT activity is also cross-regulated by protein kinases of MAPK, NF-κB, and PI3K pathways. Dysregulation of pathway may be caused by activating mutations in JAK or inactivation of SOCS.

PHYSIOLOGY
- JAK/STAT signaling mediated by JAK1–4 and STAT1–4,5A,5B,6
- STAT activity cross-regulated by MAPK, NF-κB, PI3K
- Essential in mammary gland, white blood, adipose, neuronal, cardiac, liver, stem cells
- Mediates nearly all immune regulatory processes.

NOTABLE BEHAVIORS IN CANCER
- Deregulation may be due to activating JAK mutations or inactivation of SOCS
- Deregulation may contribute to cancer, immune diseases
- Heterogeneous effects in cancer
- V617F in JAK2 seen in 50% to 95% of classical myeloproliferative neoplasms, polycythemia vera, essential thrombocytosis, primary myelofibrosis
- JAK/STAT activation in head and neck, high-grade ovarian epithelial cancers
- JAK2 amplification in gastric adenocarcinoma
- STAT1,2 drive antitumor immunity; STAT3 linked to cancer cell survival, immune suppression, and sustained inflammation in the tumor microenvironment

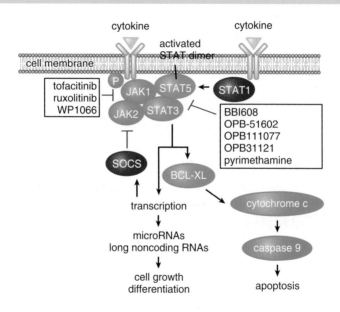

- JAK/STAT pathway transmits information through the cell membrane from chemical signals outside the cell and into genome DNA sites to regulate cell growth and differentiation.
- Many JAK/STAT pathways are important in white blood cells, mammary gland, adipocytes, neuronal cells, cardiomyocytes, hepatocytes, stem cells, and the like, and JAK/STAT deregulations may contribute to development of various diseases including immune diseases and cancers.
- There are four JAK family members (JAK1, JAK2, JAK3, and JAK4 or TYK2) and seven STAT family members (STAT1, STAT2, STAT3, STAT4, STAT5A, STAT5B, and STAT6).
- Receptor is activated by signal from cytokines (e.g., interferon, IL), growth factors, or other chemical messengers.
- After binding of ligand, cytokine receptors recruit JAKs, which phosphorylate each other and the receptor proteins, and create docking sites for STAT proteins, mostly STAT1, STAT3, and STAT5.
- STATs form dimers then translocate into nucleus. They then bind to different DNA sequence promoters, enhancers, and epigenetic regions to control transcription of target genes, microRNAs, and long noncoding RNAs and modify epigenetic markers and chromatin structures.

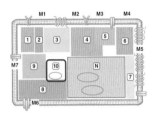

Three pathways promote Programmed Cell Death:

1. Extrinsic—TNF-Related Apoptosis-Inducing Ligand (TNF/TRAIL), FS7-associated surface antigen (FAS)
2. Intrinsic—Mitochondrial-based w/ DNA damage, ROS through BCL-2, BCL-XL, and dimers of Bax/Bak
3. CASPASE-independent pathway

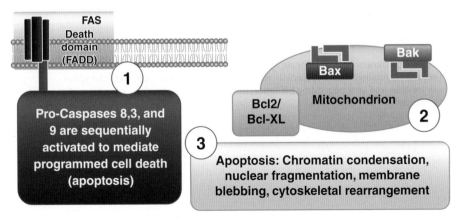

FAS
Death domain (FADD)

1

Pro-Caspases 8,3, and 9 are sequentially activated to mediate programmed cell death (apoptosis)

3

Bax
Bak
Bcl2/ Bcl-XL
Mitochondrion
2

Apoptosis: Chromatin condensation, nuclear fragmentation, membrane blebbing, cytoskeletal rearrangement

- DRs include Fas, TNFR, DR3, and DR4/5.
- After binding of ligands (e.g., FasL, TNF-α, APO-3L/TWEAK, APO-2L/TRAIL), DRs form dimers or trimers and recruit adaptor proteins that activate the caspase (casp) cascade via the mitochondria, which ultimately leads to apoptosis.
- Fas receptor (also known as apoptosis antigen 1: APO-1 or tumor necrosis factor receptor superfamily member 6 or TNFRSF6) forms the death-inducing signaling complex (DISC) as a result of ligand (FasL) binding.
- DISC is composed of the DR, adaptor protein FADD (Fas-associated protein with death domain), and caspase 8.
- TRAIL receptors 1 and 2 (TRAIL-R1 and -R2, also known as DR4 and DR5) are activated by TRAIL and also form DISC that leads to caspase cascade and apoptosis.
- DISC is inhibited by regulator FLIP (FLICE-like inhibitory protein, also known as caspase 8 and FADD-like apoptosis regulator or CFLAR).
- Other adaptor and regulator proteins mediate apoptotic signaling through different mechanisms, including RIP (receptor-interacting protein), DAXX (Fas death domain–associated xx), and ASK1 (apoptosis signal-regulating kinase 1, also known as MAP3K5).
- RIP activates BID (BH3 interacting-domain death agonist), a member of the proapoptotic BCL-2 (B-cell lymphoma 2) family.
- ASK1 is a member of the MAPKK kinase family and activates JNK (described in RAS pathway).
- Regulator proteins transport into the mitochondria and lead to a cascade of caspase activation that ultimately ends at apoptosis (PD).
- The process of apoptosis is regulated by several other signaling pathways:
  ○ AKT signaling through the inhibition of BAD
  ○ Abnormality sensor membrane detection system that responds to changes in pH or cellular damage and triggers cell death through BIM (BCL-2-like protein 11 proapoptotic regulator)
  ○ TP53 signaling through activation of BAX (BCL-2-like protein 4) proapoptotic regulator

- Proapoptotic factors act through metallothioneins (MTs), a family of proteins localized in the membrane of the Golgi apparatus that bind metals and control oxidative stress.
  - BCL-2 directly inhibits MT.
- In the absence of caspase activation, stimulation of DRs may lead to an alternative pathway of PD called necroptosis.
- Lenalidomide is a thalidomide analog and an FDA-approved inhibitor of TNF-α in multiple myeloma and mantle cell lymphoma.

NOTABLE BEHAVIORS IN CANCER
- Deregulated apoptosis linked to tumor initiation, progression, and chemoresistance
- Ligands of TNF receptors, that is, DRs, are considered as alternative to conventional chemo- or radiotherapy because of apoptotic effects independent of p53, which is often mutated in tumors.
- Some tumors are resistant to TRAIL-induced apoptosis, which is the most tumor cell–selective death mechanism.

PHYSIOLOGY
- Apoptosis is a key (silent/noninflammatory) mechanism maintaining tissue homeostasis.
- Apoptotic cells are swiftly cleared by phagocytosis to prevent release of intracellular components, which may inappropriately trigger signaling.
- DRs include Fas, TNFR, DR3, DR4/5.
- In the absence of caspase activation, DRs may trigger (inflammatory) necroptosis instead of apoptosis.

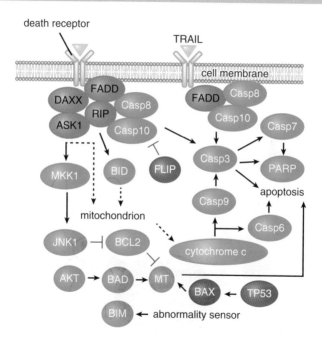

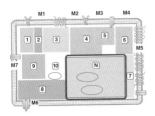

A remarkable number of factors are devoted to transcribing, controlling, and repairing DNA in order to maintain the integrity of the chromosomes, the cell cycle, and the thousands of "apps" present in every cell of the body.

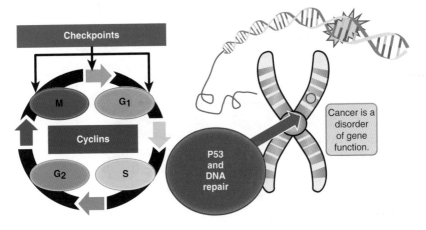

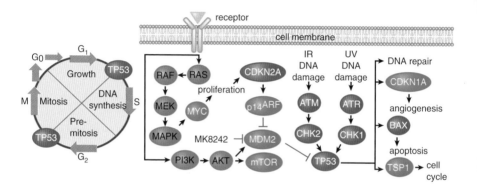

PHYSIOLOGY
- Cell cycle regulation mitigates genomic instability.
- TP53 regulates hundreds of genes and prevents genome damage.

NOTABLE BEHAVIORS IN CANCER
- Rare germline CHK2 mutations predispose to breast, colorectal cancer; somatic mutations seen in small subsets of malignancies.
- TP53 considered the most mutated genes in cancer; mutations can be inherited or somatic.
- TP53 may also be inactivated following loss of p14ARF, loss of upstream activators, loss of downstream effectors.

- *TP53* gene encodes for cellular tumor antigen (TA) or phosphoprotein p53 (name is in reference to apparent molecular mass of 53 kDa).
- Main function of TP53 is prevention of damage to genome, making it a tumor suppressor.
- TP53 acts as a transcriptional activator to several hundred genes.
- TP53 is an important regulator of G1/S and G2/M checkpoints.
- Considered the most frequently mutated gene in cancer
- Mutations may be inherited or sporadic.
- MDM2 is a negative regulator of TP53.
- MDM2 responsible for rapid turnover of TP53 (half-life 10–20 min)
  ○ MDM2 binds to TP53, blocking its transcriptional activity and initiating its transport out of the nucleus.
- MDM2 is activated by the PI3K pathway via AKT, but inhibited by RAS pathway via MYC and p14ARF.
- P14ARF is an ARF product of CDKN2A locus.
- MYC is a transcription factor that promotes proliferation by regulating the expression of specific target genes such as CDKN2A (cyclin-dependent kinase inhibitor 2A).
- Some tumors harbor amplifications of *MDM2* gene, which diminishes TP53 function.
- MDM2 inhibitors (e.g., MK-8242) are not effective against mutated TP53 because they function to silence normal TP53 function.
- Other mechanisms of TP53 inactivation include the following:
  ○ Loss of ARF (p14)
  ○ Loss of function of upstream activators including ATM and ATR, both activated by DNA double-strand breaks (DSBs)
  ○ Loss of function of downstream effectors, including angiogenesis regulator TSP1, apoptosis regulator BAX, and cell cycle regulator CDKN1A (cyclin-dependent kinase inhibitor 1A or p21)

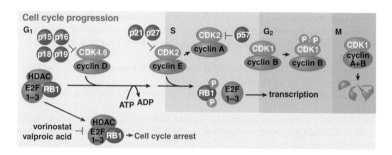

NOTABLE BEHAVIORS IN CANCER

- Loss of RB1 may result in deregulated cell proliferation.
- E2F overactivation may protect against effects of RB1 loss by inducing apoptosis.
- CDK mutation, hypermethylation, deletion are seen in various cancers.
- p15 is often deleted with p16, but may be crucial only in some leukemias.
- p57 inactivation is seen in some cancers.
- p21, p27 rarely mutated, but often downregulated; are good markers of progression and aggression.

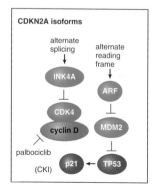

- RB1 controls transition from G1 to S phase of cell cycle by binding to E2F1, E2F2, or E2F3 proteins and thereby repressing promoters of genes needed for the entrance into S phase.
- Phosphorylation performed by CDK4/cyclin D followed by CDK2/cyclin E is needed to inactivate RB1:
  - Activities of CDK4 and CDK2 protein kinases depend on the presence of their regulatory subunits, that is, cyclin D and cyclin E, respectively.
  - Regulatory activities of these subunits fluctuate in a coordinate fashion in the course of the cell cycle.
- Loss of RB1 function upsets cell cycle regulation and may lead to unrestrained cell proliferation.
- Overactivity of E2F factor may protect against loss of RB1 function by inducing apoptosis.
- RB1/E2F complex recruits histone deacetylase (HDAC) protein, which suppresses DNA synthesis.
- HDAC inhibitors valproic acid and vorinostat are FDA-approved neuroleptics currently in clinical trials for cancer.
- Two classes of protein inhibitors of CDKs also control cell cycle:
  - CIP/KIP comprises proteins p21 (*CDKN1A* gene), p27 (*CDKN1B* gene), and p57 (*CDKN1C* gene).
  - INK comprises proteins p15 (*CDKN2B* gene), p16 (*CDKN2A* gene), p18 (*CDKN2C* gene), and p19 (*CDKN2D* gene).
- In a wide range of human cancers, *CDKN2A* gene is inactivated by mutation, hypermethylation, or deletion (regarded as tumor suppressor gene).
- CDKN2B often deleted together with CDKN2A, which may only be crucial in certain leukemia types.
- Inactivation of CDKN1C may be relevant in a small range of cancers.

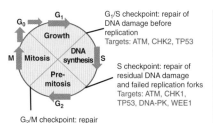

G₁/S checkpoint: repair of DNA damage before replication
Targets: ATM, CHK2, TP53

S checkpoint: repair of residual DNA damage and failed replication forks
Targets: ATM, CHK1, TP53, DNA-PK, WEE1

G₂/M checkpoint: repair of residual DNA damage before cell division
Targets: CHK1, MYT, WEE1

BRCA1,2

- Enable repair of DSBs

- Mutations in 5%–10% of all breast cancers; germline mutations in hereditary breast, ovarian cancer

- Indirectly targeted

- Therapeutic strategies quickly evolving with knowledge and understanding of DNA damage response (DDR)

DNA DAMAGE REPAIR PATHWAYS

(deficiencies drive carcinogenesis)

Damage	Damaging Agents	Repair Mechanism	Targets
Single-strand breaks	RTx Alkylating agents	Base excision	APE1 PARP
DSBs	RTx, Topo I inhibitors Nucleoside analog	Homologous recombination	ATR ATM
	RTx Topo I inhibitors	Nonhomologous end-joining	ATM DNA-PK
Bulky adducts	UV light Platinum agents	Nucleotide excision + translesion synthesis	ERCC1, XP polymerases
Substitutions insertions deletions	Replication errors Alkylating agents	Mismatch repair (MMR)	MLH, MSH MTH1, etc.

- Human cells are constantly exposed to exogenous and endogenous factors that might damage the genomic integrity and its correct transmission to the next generation.
- To respond to these threats, cells have developed an arsenal of enzymatic tools called DDR.
  - Modified bases and the DNA single-strand breaks (SSBs) are the most common form of DNA damage, and these are repaired by the base excision repair (BER) pathway.
  - For DNA DSBs, there are two major forms of repair: homologous recombination repair (HRR) and nonhomologous end-joining (NHEJ) pathways.
  - The nucleotide excision repair (NER) pathway deals with modified nucleotides that distort the structure of the double helix and it deals with UV-induced or platinum-induced DNA damage.
  - The MMR pathway deals with replication errors, including mismatch base-pairing as well as nucleotide insertions and deletions.
- DDR deficiency causes genetic aberrations that drive carcinogenesis.
- Breast cancer type 1 and type 2 (BRCA1 and BRCA2) are tumor suppressor genes that play an important role in the error-free repair of DNA DSBs, with BRCA1 also having a role in cell cycle checkpoint regulation.
- Cells with loss-of-function BRCA mutations have deficient HRR. Germline mutations in *BRCA1/2* genes are associated with hereditary breast and ovarian cancers. These mutations increase the risk of other cancers, including colon, pancreatic, and prostate. BRCA1/2 mutations account for 5% to 10% of all breast cancer cases.
- Cancer cells that have a reduced capacity to DNA repair pathway (that harbor a BRCA1 or BRCA2 mutation) are solely dependent on another, alternative pathway. This concept of synthetic lethality in cancer treatment is best demonstrated by sensitivity to poly (ADP-ribose) polymerase (PARP) inhibitors that are effective in patients with BRCA1/BRCA2-mutated cancers.

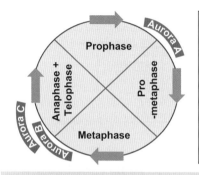

PHYSIOLOGY
- Regulates events in mitosis, including chromosome segregation, spindle checkpoint
- Aurora A required for centrosome function; expression regulated by p53; interacts with BRCA1
- Aurora B required for attachment of mitotic spindle to centromere; phosphorylates histone-H3; function regulated/modified by topoisomerase II, survivin, borealin, INCENP
- In mutually antagonistic relationship with TP53

NOTABLE BEHAVIORS IN CANCER

- Defects in chromosome segregation promote genetic instability, cell cycle progression, deregulated proliferation, tumorigenesis
- Mutated or amplified in cancer cells; diffusely distributed rather than concentrated at specific subcellular structures
- Overexpressed in cancer stem cells
- Stabilize MYC, reinforcing its tumorigenic properties
- Mutations in chromosome 20q13, which spans Aurora A, linked to poor prognosis
- Aurora A overexpression associated with poorer prognosis in specific cancers, predictive of distant metastasis in triple-negative breast cancer, others
- Aurora A variants Phe31/Ile and 91A-169G haplotype predict poor response to cisplatin-based therapy

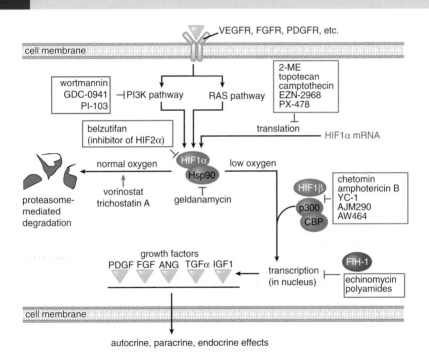

- Angiogenesis is a hallmark of cancer represented by the development of new blood vessels to keep up with the tumor needs, a process that is tightly controlled by pro- and antiangiogenic chemical signals.
- The **angiogenic switch** occurs when, in the hypoxic and inflammatory context of cancer, proangiogenic signals outweigh antiangiogenic signals, leading to tumor neovascularization. The shift in balance toward proangiogenic signals favors the abnormal and rapid growth and proliferation of local blood vessels.
- The sprouting of new blood vessels from the existing vasculature is the most widely investigated mode of new vessel formation in tumors. There are five other mechanisms of new vessel recruitment:
  - Vasculogenesis involves vessel formation by endothelial progenitor cells (EPCs), which are recruited from the bone marrow and/or are resident in vascular walls.
  - Intussusception is the splitting of preexisting vessels to give rise to daughter vessels.
  - Vessel co-option occurs when cancer cells grow around and co-opt the existing vasculature.
  - Vascular mimicry is a process in which cancer cells get incorporated into the blood vessel wall.
  - Tumor stem cell to EC differentiation occurs when cancer stem cell–like cells differentiate into ECs.
- Tumor angiogenesis, which allows for continued tumor growth, is often a deregulated process that results in incomplete, irregular, tortuous, and leaky capillaries. Tumor vessels exhibit bidirectional blood flow, are not constantly perfused, and tend to be larger than normal vessels with an altered surface area-to-volume ratio that results in poor nutrient delivery and waste removal.

Tumor hypoxia and inflammation trigger a proangiogenic switch that overcomes normal antiangiogenic mechanisms.

Angiogenic Switch

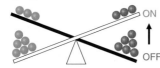

Activators, *e.g.,*	Inhibitors, *e.g.,*
● HIF-1α	● angiostatin
● cytokines (IL-8)	● tumstatin
● growth factors	● endostatin
● inflammation	● TSP-1
	● TP53

(Modified from Hanahan D, Folkman J. Patterns and emerging mechanisms of the angiogenic switch during tumorigenesis. *Cell.* 1996;86:353–364. With permission from Elsevier.)

Angiogenic Effects Of Genetic Lesions

Gain of Function: Oncogenes		
PI3K	↑VEGF	↓TSP-1
HRAS	↑VEGF	
EGFR	↑VEGF, ↑FGF, ↑IL-8	
ERBB2	↑VEGF	
BCL2	↑VEGF	
SRC	↑VEGF	↓TSP-1
FOS	↑VEGF	
Loss of Function: Tumor Suppressors		
TP53	↑VEGF	↓TSP-1
VHL	↑VEGF	
PTEN	↑VEGF	
RB		↓TSP-1

Adapted from Wicki A, Christofori G. The angiogenic switch in tumorigenesis. In: Marmé D, Fusenig N, eds. *Tumor Angiogenesis: Basic Mechanisms and Cancer Therapy.* Springer; 2008:73.

NEW TUMOR VESSELS FORM BY

- Co-opting of existing vessels
- Differentiation of EPCs into new vessels
- Differentiation of cancer stem cell–like cells into ECs
- Incorporation of cancer cells into vessel walls
- Splitting of/sprouting from existing vessels

- Hypoxia or low oxygen tension results from uncontrolled proliferation of cancer cells in the absence of a functional and adequate vascular bed. It is a major driver of tumor angiogenesis.
  - The 2019 Nobel Prize was awarded to William Kaelin Jr., Sir Peter Ratcliffe, and Gregg Semenza for elucidating the importance of hypoxia-induced factors that respond to changes in oxygen levels.
  - Under normoxic conditions, hypoxia-inducible transcription factor-1 alpha (HIF-1α) subunits are subjected to von Hippel–Lindau (VHL)-directed protein degradation. VHL itself is a tumor suppressor, and VHL mutations have been implicated in malignancies such as renal cell carcinoma.
- Hypoxic conditions stabilize HIF-1α, allowing it to translocate to the nucleus and, along with HIF-1β, initiate the transcription of proangiogenic genes such as VEGF. Examples of proangiogenic signals secreted by tumors include the following:
  - Growth factors such as FGF, ANG, PDGF, VEGF
  - Cytokines such as IL-8
- TP53 negatively regulates angiogenesis by downregulating VEGF and other proangiogenic factors while increasing the expression of antiangiogenic signals such as thrombospondin 1 (TSP1). Loss of P53 function promotes VEGF expression and tumor angiogenesis, although the underlying mechanisms remain unclear and controversial.
- Other examples of endogenous inhibitors of angiogenesis include angiostatin, endostatin, tumstatin, and camstatin.

Immunotherapy

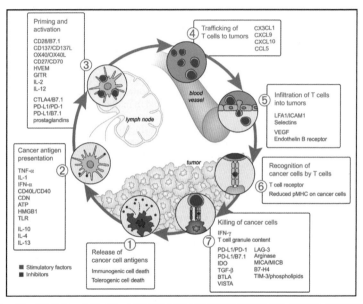

(Reprinted from Chen DS, Mellman I. Oncology meets immunology: the cancer-immunity cycle. *Immunity*. 2013;39(1):1–10. With permission from Elsevier.)

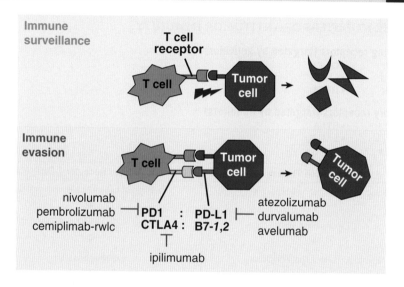

OTHER MODIFIERS OF ANTITUMOR IMMUNITY

Activating receptors (targeted by activators)
- 41BB
- CD28
- GITR
- OX40
- CD27
- HVEM

Inhibitory receptors (targeted by inhibitors)
- VISTA
- TIM-3
- BTLA
- LAG-3

Adoptive Cell Therapy	Chimeric Antigen Receptor T Cells (CAR-T)
Isolation of tumor-infiltrating lymphocytes (TILs)	Isolation of native T cells from patient
↓	↓
Expansion in vitro	Genetic engineering to express CAR
↓	↓
Reinfusion after lymphodepletion	Expansion in vitro
	↓
	Reinfusion

PD-1/PD-L1

- PD-1 is a cell surface protein involved in downregulating T-cell response, preventing autoimmunity under normal conditions.
- PD-1 is typically expressed on T cells and has two ligands, PD-L1 and PD-L2. Interactions between PD-1 and PD-L1 result in T-cell downregulation, impairment, exhaustion, and apoptosis, all of which lead to immune evasion. By hyperexpressing PD-L1, certain cancers can thwart the host immune system.

CTLA-4

- Cytotoxic T-lymphocyte antigen 4 (CTLA-4) is a receptor found exclusively on T cells. Activation of CTLA-4 downregulates T-cell activation and therefore immune response.
- CD80 (B7-1) and CD86 (B7-2) are ligands for CTLA-4, which when bound to each other prevent T-cell activation and immune signaling. Antibodies inhibiting CTLA-4, therefore, promote activation of effector T cells and downregulation of T regulatory cells (Tregs).
- When compared with PD1/PD-L1 blockade, CTLA-4 inhibition generally creates more immune-related toxicities. Where PD1/PD-L1–directed therapies depend on interaction of tumor and T cells, blocking CTLA-4 upregulates the earlier stages of T-cell activation and is independent of tumor interaction.

GITR

- Glucocorticoid-induced TNF receptor (GITR) is a receptor that belongs to the TNF receptor family, like OX-40 and 4-1BB. It is a costimulatory receptor that is highly expressed on Tregs, but is also found on T-effector cells, NK cells, macrophages, and dendritic cells. The ligand for GITR (GITRL) is expressed on antigen-presenting cells.

- Modulation of the GITR and GITRL results in intratumoral Treg inhibition and expansion of cytotoxic and memory CD8+ T cells.
- Antibodies to GITR or GITRL fusion proteins are in the early clinical phases of development and are being evaluated in solid tumors.
- Current clinical trials are evaluating GITR/GITRL modulation in combination with PD-1 or CTLA-4 inhibitors.

4-1BB

- 4-1BB (CD137) is a receptor that belongs to the TNF receptor family, like OX-40 and GITR. It is expressed on multiple immune cells with its downstream effect being activating and upregulating cytotoxic T cells. There is some evidence to suggest that activation of 4-1BB enhances antibody-dependent cell-mediated cytotoxicity (ADCC).
- There are currently two 4-1BB monoclonal antibodies being investigated—urelumab, a fully humanized immunoglobulin G (IgG)4, and utomilumab, a fully humanized IgG2—both of which are being investigated in clinical trials as a single agent and in combination with other immune checkpoint inhibitors.
- Although 4-1BB targeted therapies have a high potential for antitumor effect, there have been severe adverse immune-related events including hematologic toxicity and hepatitis.

OX40

- OX40 (CD134) is a costimulatory receptor that belongs to the TNF receptor family, like 4-1BB and GITR. It is expressed on T cells following their activation and promotes their survival during immune response.

- Modulation of OX40 or its ligand (OX40L) results in expansion and promotion of cytotoxic CD8+ T cells alongside nonregulatory CD4+ T cells.
- Several clinical trials with OX40 agonists are in clinical trials mostly in combination with PD1/PD-L1 and CTLA-4 inhibitors.

LAG3

- Lymphocyte activation gene 3 (*LAG-3*) (CD223) is a surface protein expressed on activated T cells, B cells, NK cells, and dendritic cells. LAG-3 is similar in structure to CD4 and binds to MHC Class II.
- LAG-3 functions as an immune checkpoint, and its interaction with MHC Class II inhibits downstream effects on CD4+ T cells. Increased LAG-3 expression on tumor samples has been identified in colorectal cancer and melanoma. By increasing LAG-3 expression, cancer cells can evade immune recognition and destruction.
- Blockade of LAG-3 leads to activation of T cells and inhibition of Tregs and upregulation of T-cell proliferation.
- LAG-3 antibodies are being investigated alone and in combination with PD-1 inhibitors.

TIM-3

- T-cell immunoglobulin mucin-3 (TIM-3) is a receptor expressed on a variety of cells including T cells, Tregs, NK cells, and dendritic cells. TIM-3+ T cells are considered dysfunctional and exhausted.
- TIM-3 functions as an immune checkpoint similar to, and possibly in conjunction with, PD-1.
- Patients previously failing PD-1 inhibitors have developed immune escape by upregulating TIM-3 as a response.

TIGIT

- T-cell immunoreceptor with Ig and ITIM domains (TIGIT) interacts with CD155 to suppress T cells and NKs, thereby inhibiting immune reactions, for example, antitumor immunity.
- Overexpressed on TA-specific CD8+ T cells and CD8+ TILs from patients with melanoma, breast cancer, non–small-cell lung carcinoma, colon adenocarcinoma, gastric cancer, acute myeloid leukemia, and multiple myeloma
- Dual blockade of TIGIT and PD-1 leads to increased cell proliferation, cytokine production, and degranulation of TA-specific CD8+ T cells and TIL CD8+ T cells.

ADOPTIVE CELL THERAPY

- Cell therapy involves the infusion of autologous or allogeneic immune cells used to target cancer cells.
- TILs were first used in the treatment of melanoma. TILs are essentially host immune cells that are isolated from the patient's own tumor sample. The TILs are expanded in vitro to a prespecified cell count and infused into the same patient after having received lympho-depleting chemotherapy. Patients have attained sustained complete response using TILs, and trials are ongoing.
- CAR-T use genetically altered autologous T cells that target certain antigens. The patient's native T cells are obtained peripherally through lymphopheresis. They are then genetically altered using a variety of different techniques to express a CAR. Once the CAR-T is generated, it is expanded in vitro and eventually infused back into a patient that has received lympho-depleting chemotherapy.
- CAR-T can target a variety of antigens, but the most common in development has been the B-cell antigen CD19.
- The use of CAR-T is being investigated in solid tumors with targets including EGFR, HER2, CEA, MSLN, PSMA, and CA125.

THYROID FUNCTION

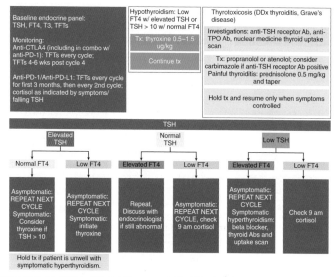

Baseline endocrine panel: TSH, FT4, T3, TFTs

Monitoring:
Anti-CTLA4 (including in combo w/ anti-PD-1): TFTs every cycle; TFTs 4-6 wks post cycle 4

Anti-PD-1/Anti-PD-L1: TFTs every cycle for first 3 months, then every 2nd cycle; cortisol as indicated by symptoms/ falling TSH

Hypothyroidism: Low FT4 w/ elevated TSH or TSH > 10 w/ normal FT4

Tx: thyroxine 0.5–1.5 ug/kg

Continue tx

Thyrotoxicosis (DDx thyroiditis, Grave's disease)

Investigations: anti-TSH receptor Ab, anti-TPO Ab, nuclear medicine thyroid uptake scan

Tx: propranolol or atenolol; consider carbimazole if anti-TSH receptor Ab positive Painful thyroiditis: prednisolone 0.5 mg/kg and taper

Hold tx and resume only when symptoms controlled

TSH

Elevated TSH — Normal TSH — Low TSH

Normal FT4 | Low FT4 | Elevated FT4 | Low FT4 | Elevated FT4 | Low FT4

Asymptomatic: REPEAT NEXT CYCLE Symptomatic: Consider thyroxine if TSH > 10

Asymptomatic: REPEAT NEXT CYCLE Symptomatic: initiate thyroxine

Repeat, Discuss with endocrinologist if still abnormal

Asymptomatic: REPEAT NEXT CYCLE, check 9 am cortisol

Asymptomatic: REPEAT NEXT CYCLE Symptomatic hyperthyroidism: beta blocker, thyroid Abs and uptake scan

Check 9 am cortisol

Hold tx if patient is unwell with symptomatic hyperthyroidism.

(Data from Haanen J, Carbonnel F, Robert C, et al. Management of toxicities from immunotherapy: ESMO Clinical Practice Guidelines for diagnosis, treatment and follow-up. *Ann Oncol.* 2017;28:iv119–iv142.)

DIARRHEA AND COLITIS

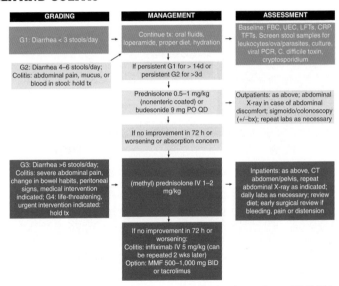

GRADING	MANAGEMENT	ASSESSMENT
G1: Diarrhea < 3 stools/day	Continue tx: oral fluids, loperamide, proper diet, hydration	Baseline: FBC, UEC, LFTs, CRP, TFTs. Screen stool samples for leukocytes/ova/parasites, culture, viral PCR, C. difficile toxin, cryptosporidium
G2: Diarrhea 4–6 stools/day; Colitis: abdominal pain, mucus, or blood in stool: hold tx	If persistent G1 for > 14d or persistent G2 for >3d → Prednisolone 0.5–1 mg/kg (nonenteric coated) or budesonide 9 mg PO QD → If no improvement in 72 h or worsening or absorption concern	Outpatients: as above; abdominal X-ray in case of abdominal discomfort; sigmoido/colonoscopy (+/–bx); repeat labs as necessary
G3: Diarrhea >6 stools/day; Colitis: severe abdominal pain, change in bowel habits, peritoneal signs, medical intervention indicated; G4: life-threatening, urgent intervention indicated: hold tx	(methyl) prednisolone IV 1–2 mg/kg → If no improvement in 72 h or worsening: Colitis: infliximab IV 5 mg/kg (can be repeated 2 wks later) Option: MMF 500–1,000 mg BID or tacrolimus	Inpatients: as above, CT abdomen/pelvis, repeat abdominal X-ray as indicated; daily labs as necessary; review diet; early surgical review if bleeding, pain or distension

(Data from Haanen J, Carbonnel F, Robert C, et al. Management of toxicities from immunotherapy: ESMO Clinical Practice Guidelines for diagnosis, treatment and follow-up. *Ann Oncol*. 2017;28:iv119–iv142.)

HEPATITIS

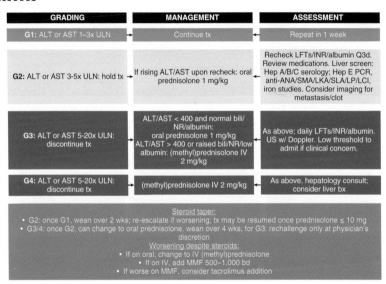

GRADING	MANAGEMENT	ASSESSMENT
G1: ALT or AST 1–3x ULN	Continue tx	Repeat in 1 week
G2: ALT or AST 3-5x ULN: hold tx	If rising ALT/AST upon recheck: oral prednisolone 1 mg/kg	Recheck LFTs/INR/albumin Q3d. Review medications. Liver screen: Hep A/B/C serology; Hep E PCR, anti-ANA/SMA/LKA/SLA/LP/LCI, iron studies. Consider imaging for metastasis/clot
G3: ALT or AST 5-20x ULN: discontinue tx	ALT/AST < 400 and normal bili/NR/albumin: oral prednisolone 1 mg/kg. ALT/AST > 400 or raised bili/NR/low albumin: (methyl)prednisolone IV 2 mg/kg	As above; daily LFTs/INR/albumin. US w/ Doppler. Low threshold to admit if clinical concern.
G4: ALT or AST 5-20x ULN: discontinue tx	(methyl)prednisolone IV 2 mg/kg	As above, hepatology consult; consider liver bx

Steroid taper:
- G2: once G1, wean over 2 wks; re-escalate if worsening; tx may be resumed once prednisolone ≤ 10 mg
- G3/4: once G2, can change to oral prednisolone, wean over 4 wks; for G3: rechallenge only at physician's discretion

Worsening despite steroids:
- If on oral, change to IV (methyl)prednisolone
- If on IV, add MMF 500–1,000 bd
- If worse on MMF, consider tacrolimus addition

(Data from Haanen J, Carbonnel F, Robert C, et al. Management of toxicities from immunotherapy: ESMO Clinical Practice Guidelines for diagnosis, treatment and follow-up. *Ann Oncol.* 2017;28:iv119–iv142.)

PERIPHERAL NEUROLOGIC TOXICITY

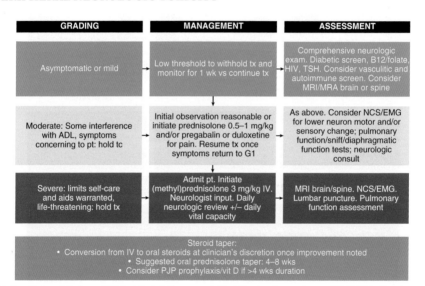

GRADING	MANAGEMENT	ASSESSMENT
Asymptomatic or mild	Low threshold to withhold tx and monitor for 1 wk vs continue tx	Comprehensive neurologic exam. Diabetic screen, B12/folate, HIV, TSH. Consider vasculitic and autoimmune screen. Consider MRI/MRA brain or spine
Moderate: Some interference with ADL, symptoms concerning to pt: hold tc	Initial observation reasonable or initiate prednisolone 0.5–1 mg/kg and/or pregabalin or duloxetine for pain. Resume tx once symptoms return to G1	As above. Consider NCS/EMG for lower neuron motor and/or sensory change; pulmonary function/sniff/diaphragmatic function tests; neurologic consult
Severe: limits self-care and aids warranted, life-threatening: hold tx	Admit pt. Initiate (methyl)prednisolone 3 mg/kg IV. Neurologist input. Daily neurologic review +/– daily vital capacity	MRI brain/spine. NCS/EMG. Lumbar puncture. Pulmonary function assessment

Steroid taper:
- Conversion from IV to oral steroids at clinician's discretion once improvement noted
- Suggested oral prednisolone taper: 4–8 wks
- Consider PJP prophylaxis/vit D if >4 wks duration

(Data from Haanen J, Carbonnel F, Robert C, et al. Management of toxicities from immunotherapy: ESMO Clinical Practice Guidelines for diagnosis, treatment and follow-up. *Ann Oncol.* 2017;28:iv119–iv142.)

PNEUMONITIS

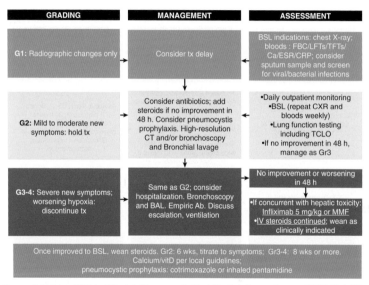

GRADING	MANAGEMENT	ASSESSMENT
G1: Radiographic changes only	Consider tx delay	BSL indications: chest X-ray; bloods : FBC/LFTs/TFTs/Ca/ESR/CRP; consider sputum sample and screen for viral/bacterial infections
G2: Mild to moderate new symptoms: hold tx	Consider antibiotics; add steroids if no improvement in 48 h. Consider pneumocystis prophylaxis. High-resolution CT and/or bronchoscopy and Bronchial lavage	• Daily outpatient monitoring • BSL (repeat CXR and bloods weekly) • Lung function testing including TCLO • If no improvement in 48 h, manage as Gr3
G3-4: Severe new symptoms; worsening hypoxia: discontinue tx	Same as G2; consider hospitalization. Bronchoscopy and BAL. Empiric Ab. Discuss escalation, ventilation	No improvement or worsening in 48 h • If concurrent with hepatic toxicity: Infliximab 5 mg/kg or MMF • IV steroids continued; wean as clinically indicated

Once improved to BSL, wean steroids. Gr2: 6 wks, titrate to symptoms; Gr3-4: 8 wks or more. Calcium/vitD per local guidelines; pneumocystic prophylaxis: cotrimoxazole or inhaled pentamidine

(Data from Haanen J, Carbonnel F, Robert C, et al. Management of toxicities from immunotherapy: ESMO Clinical Practice Guidelines for diagnosis, treatment and follow-up. *Ann Oncol*. 2017;28:iv119–iv142.)

NEPHRITIS

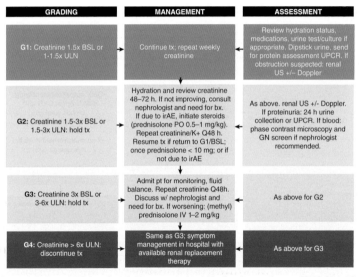

GRADING	MANAGEMENT	ASSESSMENT
G1: Creatinine 1.5x BSL or 1-1.5x ULN	Continue tx; repeat weekly creatinine	Review hydration status, medications, urine test/culture if appropriate. Dipstick urine, send for protein assessment UPCR. If obstruction suspected: renal US +/– Doppler
G2: Creatinine 1.5-3x BSL or 1.5-3x ULN: hold tx	Hydration and review creatinine 48–72 h. If not improving, consult nephrologist and need for bx. If due to irAE, initiate steroids (prednisolone PO 0.5–1 mg/kg). Repeat creatinine/K+ Q48 h. Resume tx if return to G1/BSL; once prednisolone < 10 mg; or if not due to irAE	As above. renal US +/– Doppler. If proteinuria: 24 h urine collection or UPCR. If blood: phase contrast microscopy and GN screen if nephrologist recommended.
G3: Creatinine 3x BSL or 3-6x ULN: hold tx	Admit pt for monitoring, fluid balance. Repeat creatinine Q48h. Discuss w/ nephrologist and need for bx. If worsening: (methyl) prednisolone IV 1–2 mg/kg	As above for G2
G4: Creatinine > 6x ULN: discontinue tx	Same as G3; symptom management in hospital with available renal replacement therapy	As above for G3

(Data from Haanen J, Carbonnel F, Robert C, et al. Management of toxicities from immunotherapy: ESMO Clinical Practice Guidelines for diagnosis, treatment and follow-up. *Ann Oncol.* 2017;28:iv119–iv142.)

SKIN RASH/TOXICITY

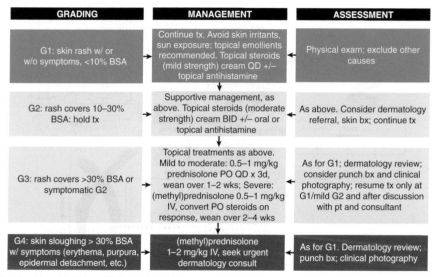

GRADING	MANAGEMENT	ASSESSMENT
G1: skin rash w/ or w/o symptoms, <10% BSA	Continue tx. Avoid skin irritants, sun exposure; topical emollients recommended. Topical steroids (mild strength) cream QD +/− topical antihistamine	Physical exam; exclude other causes
G2: rash covers 10–30% BSA: hold tx	Supportive management, as above. Topical steroids (moderate strength) cream BID +/− oral or topical antihistamine	As above. Consider dermatology referral, skin bx; continue tx
G3: rash covers >30% BSA or symptomatic G2	Topical treatments as above. Mild to moderate: 0.5–1 mg/kg prednisolone PO QD x 3d, wean over 1–2 wks; Severe: (methyl)prednisolone 0.5–1 mg/kg IV, convert PO steroids on response, wean over 2–4 wks	As for G1; dermatology review; consider punch bx and clinical photography; resume tx only at G1/mild G2 and after discussion with pt and consultant
G4: skin sloughing > 30% BSA w/ symptoms (erythema, purpura, epidermal detachment, etc.)	(methyl)prednisolone 1–2 mg/kg IV, seek urgent dermatology consult	As for G1. Dermatology review; punch bx; clinical photography

(Data from Haanen J, Carbonnel F, Robert C, et al. Management of toxicities from immunotherapy: ESMO Clinical Practice Guidelines for diagnosis, treatment and follow-up. *Ann Oncol.* 2017;28:iv119–iv142.)

HERITABLE GENOMIC CHANGES NOT CAUSED BY CHANGES IN DNA SEQUENCE

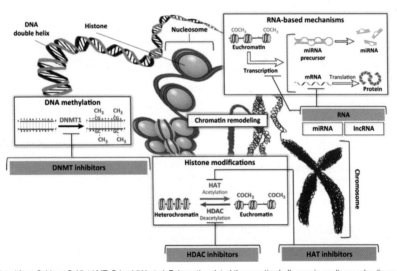

(Reprinted from Schiano C, Vietri MT, Grimaldi V, et al. Epigenetic-related therapeutic challenges in cardiovascular disease. *Trends Pharmacol Sci*. 2015;36:226–235. With permission from Elsevier.)

- **Epigenetics** are defined as heritable changes in the genome that are not caused by alterations in DNA sequence. The DNA exists in the form of chromatin, which is composed of units of nucleosomes. Nucleosome contains an octamer of histone core and the wrapping DNA of 147 bp.
- **Epigenetic mechanisms** include the DNA methylation, histone posttranslational modification, nucleosome restructure, and noncoding RNAs. These mechanisms regulate the switch between the active "euchromatic" and the suppressive "heterochromatic" transcription states.
  - **DNA methylation** involves the covalent transfer of a methyl group to the C-5 position of the cytosine ring of DNA by DNA methyltransferase (DNMT). In cancer cells, DNAs are globally hypomethylated but locally hypermethylated at the promoters of tumor suppressor genes. DNMT is overexpressed in many cancer types including leukemia and lung, breast, gastric, and colorectal cancers.
  - **DNMT inhibitors** azacitidine and decitabine are approved by the FDA for myelodysplastic syndrome. In clinical trials, low doses of DNMT inhibitors are used to sensitize cancer cells to radiation therapy, chemotherapy, and immunotherapies.
- **Histone modifications** are posttranscriptional modifications of the histones in a highly dynamic manner, mainly including histone acetylation, methylation, phosphorylation, ubiquitylation, and sumoylation.
- **Histone modifiers** respond to the upstream signals, recognize and bind (readers) to specific histone regions, and catalytically modify (writers or erasers) histone residues. Many of these modifications are abnormally regulated in cancer.

- **Histone acetylation** occurs on lysine residues on the histone tail and is associated with transcription activation. It is catalyzed by competing enzymes such as histone lysine acetyltransferases (HATs) and HDACs.
- **HDAC inhibitors** induce reexpression of tumor suppressors such as p21, p53, and NF-κB. Vorinostat, belinostat, and romidepsin are FDA-approved HDAC inhibitors for T-cell lymphoma. Panobinostat is another FDA-approved HDAC inhibitor in treating multiple myeloma.
- **Bromodomain and extraterminal protein (BET)** is a subfamily of bromodomains, which are histone acetylation readers. BET is a key player in transcriptional elongation and cell cycle progression. **BET inhibitors** have shown antitumor effects in NUT-midline carcinoma and hematologic malignancies in clinical trials.
- **Histone methylation** occurs on arginine and lysine residues and may either activate or inactivate transcription.
  - **EZH2** is the catalytic subunit of PRC2 complex, which trimethylates H3K27. High activity of EZH2 results in alterations in cell self-renewal and differentiation, cell cycle progression, and DNA repair. **EZH2 inhibitors** show antitumor and synthetic lethal effects with deficiency of SWI/SNF chromatin remodeling complexes.
  - **PRMT5**, a histone methyltransferase, is overexpressed in AML, lymphomas, glioblastomas, and lung and ovarian cancers. **PRMT5 inhibitors** are being tested in treating non-Hodgkin lymphoma and other solid tumors in clinical trials.
  - **Histone lysine demethylase LSD1** demethylates H3K4 and H3K9. **LSD1 inhibitors** induce apoptosis and prodifferentiation in leukemia cells in preclinical studies and are being tested in clinical trials.
- **Chromatin remodeling** uses the energy from ATP hydrolysis to mobilize and exchange histones, and thus allows open chromatin for gene activation. It is regulated by families of SWI/SNF, ISWI, and NuRD/Mi-2/CHD. The components of SWI/SNF family are tumor suppressors, for example, SNF5 loss leads to the development of malignant rhabdoid tumors. SWI/SNF deficiency is combined with other antitumor agents to reach therapeutic synthetic lethality in clinical trials.

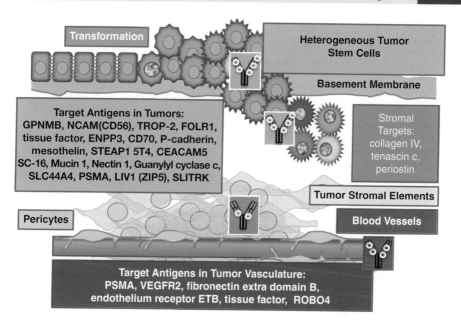

- Antibody–drug conjugates (ADCs) are a hybrid of cytotoxic drug and specific antibody joined by a linker.
- They provide targeted delivery of a cytotoxic agent with a reduced amount of toxicity.
- Their efficacy depends not on a mutation in the genome, but on a suitable marker on the cell surface.
- A successful ADC depends on a firmly attached cell surface antigen for the antibody to bind.
- These target antigens should be expressed at higher levels on tumor than on normal cells. Drug uptake should be via receptor-mediated endocytosis.
- Patients tend to benefit proportionally to the level of antigen expression on tumor cells.
- ADC specificity is limited because of the bystander effect, which causes cell death in adjacent cells that did not internalize the drug.
- Alternatively, ADCs can target the stroma and vasculature rather than the tumor itself.
- Commonly, the antibody portion is a human IgG1, which has the occasional benefit of activating antibody-dependent cellular cytotoxicity.
- The linker is a crucial piece of an ADC because it must not release the toxin in the bloodstream, while also releasing when necessary after endocytosis. The linker usually holds multiple molecules of a toxin to provide adequate cellular kill, with an optimal ratio of four toxin molecules to one antibody.
- Linker can be cleavable or noncleavable, with both approaches successfully used in drug development. (T-DM1 is a noncleavable linker.)
- The cytotoxic payload must be highly potent even at nanomolar concentrations, making traditional chemotherapy ineffective.
- Microtubule inhibitors such as auristatins cause G2/M-cell cycle arrest (brentuximab–vedotin).
- DNA-damaging agents such as calicheamicin work throughout the cell cycle (inotuzumab–ozogamicin).

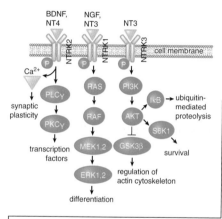

PHYSIOLOGY

- Neurotrophin receptors that regulate neuronal development and function; as well as memory, body weight, appetite, proprioception, pain, thermal regulation

NOTABLE BEHAVIORS IN CANCER

- Activation of downstream pathways drives tumor growth.
- Gene fusions pathognomonic in rare cancers such as congenital fibrosarcoma, secretory breast cancer, mammary analogue secretory carcinoma (MASC) of salivary gland
- Fusion partners include TPR, ETV6, TP53, TFG
- Mutations, splice variants, and overexpression also potentially tumorigenic
- Fusions also seen in papillary thyroid carcinoma (12%–14.5%), lung adenocarcinoma (3.3%), Spitzoid neoplasms (16%), pediatric high-grade glioma (40%)
- Highly responsive to first-generation inhibitors, but eventually acquire resistance, most commonly through solvent front mutations; resistance can be overcome by second-generation inhibitors currently in clinical trials; NGS needed to identify resistance mutations postprogression/nonresponse

- The tropomyosin-related kinases (TRKs) are neurotrophin receptors from the tyrosine kinase family and consist of three members: TRKA, TRKB, and TRKC, which are encoded by *NTRK1*, *NTRK2*, and *NTRK3* genes. The corresponding in vivo ligands are as follows: TRKA—neurotrophic growth factor (NGF) and neurotrophin-3 (NT-3); TRKB—brain-derived neurotrophic factor (BDNF) and neurotrophin-4 (NT-4); TRKC—NT-3 (Amatu et al., 2016).
- The TRK receptor family is involved in neuronal development, including the growth and function of neuronal synapses. In adults, TRK receptors regulate memory, body weight, appetite, proprioception, pain, and thermal regulation.
- Tropomyosin sequences cause activation of the kinase activity of the receptor with downstream activation of MAPK, PI3K, and PLCg pathways, resulting in cell proliferation, increased cell survival, and migration leading to tumor growth.
- Gene fusions involving the NTRK family are pathognomonic in rare cancers such as congenital fibrosarcoma, secretory breast cancer, and MASC of the salivary gland.
- *NTRK* gene fusions have been described across several cancer types with varying frequencies such as the following:
  - Papillary thyroid carcinoma (NTRK1—12%; NTRK3—14.5%)
  - Lung adenocarcinoma (3.3%)
  - Spitzoid neoplasms (16%)
  - Pediatric high-grade glioma (40%)

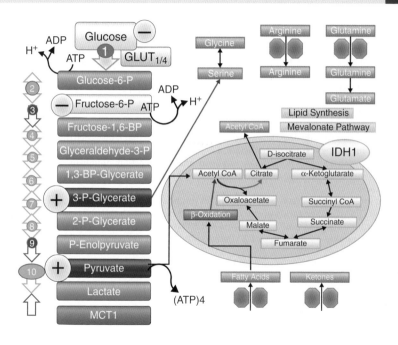

- Tumor cells metabolize glucose, lactate, pyruvate, hydroxybutyrate, acetate, glutamine, arginine, and fatty acids at much higher rates than nontumor tissue.
- These intermediary metabolites are released by catabolic cells, taken up by tumor cells, and used to replenish TCA-cycle intermediates and to fuel oxidative phosphorylation (reverse Warburg effect).
- Enasidenib (formerly AG-221) is a first-in-class inhibitor of mutated isocitrate dehydrogenase 2 (IDH2) and is now FDA-approved to treat acute myeloid leukemia.
- Similarly, ivosidenib, an inhibitor of IDH1, is FDA-approved in cholangiocarcinoma. The IDH enzyme normally metabolizes isocitrate into α-ketoglutarate. When mutated, it also converts α-ketoglutarate into 2-hydroxyglutarate, an oncometabolite that causes cell differentiation defects by impairing histone demethylation.
- Targeting glycolysis, mitochondrial metabolism, and amino acid metabolism with drug combinations holds promise as an antitumor strategy, and the following drugs are in early-phase trials:
  - Drugs inhibiting glycolysis—silibinin (GLUT1 inhibitor) (Ooi and Gomperts, 2015), TLN-232 (inhibits PKM2 dimerization and activity) (Vander Heiden et al., 2010)
  - Drugs inhibiting glutamine metabolism—CB-839 (Gross et al., 2014) and bis-2-(5-phenylacetamido-1,2,4-thiadiazol-2-yl)ethyl sulfide (BPTES) (Xiang et al., 2015) (glutaminase inhibitors)
  - Drugs targeting lactate, pyruvate, and acetyl-CoA production—AZD3965 (MCT1 inhibitor) (Polański et al., 2014)
  - Drugs degrading circulating arginine—ADI-PEG20 (Ascierto et al., 2005)

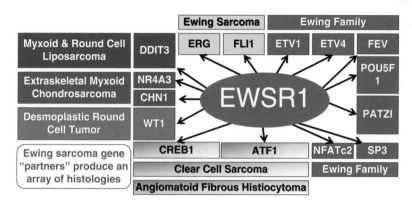

ATF1, cyclic AMP (cAMP)–dependent **T**ranscription **F**actor **1**; **CHN1**, **CH**imaerin **N**ervous system **1** protein gene; CREB1, cAMP **R**esponsive **E**lement–**B**inding protein **1**; **DDIT3**, **D**NA **D**amage Inducible **T**ranscript **3** gene; **ERG**, **E**rythroblast transformation factor–**R**elated **G**ene; **ETV1**, **ETS V**ariant **1**; **ETV4**, **E**-Twenty-six **T**ranslocation **V**ariant **4**; **FEV**, **F**ifth **E**wing **V**ariant protein (ETS oncogene family); **FLI1**, **F**riend **L**eukemia **I**ntegration **1** gene; **NFATC2**, **N**uclear **F**actor of **A**ctivated **T** **C**ells **2**; **NR4A3**, **N**uclear (hormone) **R**eceptor member **4A3**; **PATZ1**, **P**OZ/BTB and **AT** Hook–Containing **Z**inc Finger **1**; **POU5F1**, Protein coding **POU** class **5** homeobox **1** gene; **SP3**, GT/GC box promoter transcription factor gene; **WT1**, **W**ilms **T**umor protein coding gene **1**.

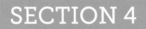

Targeted and Immunotherapy Agents

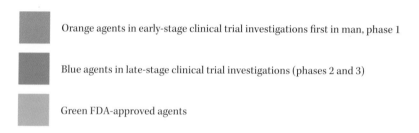

Orange agents in early-stage clinical trial investigations first in man, phase 1

Blue agents in late-stage clinical trial investigations (phases 2 and 3)

Green FDA-approved agents

- 17-AAG: 17-allylaminogeldanamycin
- 2HG: 2-hydroxyglutarate
- 5FU: 5-fluorouracil
- ADCC: antibody-dependent cell-mediated cytotoxicity
- AICARFT: aminoimidazole carboxamide ribonucleotide formyltransferase
- ALK: anaplastic lymphoma kinase
- ALT: alanine transaminase
- AML: acute myelogenous leukemia
- AR: androgen receptor
- AST: aspartate aminotransferase
- ATM: ataxia telangiectasia mutated
- AURKA: Aurora A kinase
- AURKB: Aurora B kinase
- BCRP: breast cancer resistance protein
- BNP: brain natriuretic peptide
- BRCA: BReast CAncer susceptibility gene
- BTK: Bruton's tyrosine kinase
- CAR: chimeric antigen receptor
- CBP: CREB-binding protein
- CCR4: CC chemokine receptor 4
- CD: cytosine deaminase
- CDK: cyclin-dependent kinase
- CLL: chronic lymphocytic leukemia
- CMV: cytomegalovirus
- CPK: creatine phosphokinase

- CREB: cAMP response element-binding protein
- CTCL: cutaneous T-cell lymphoma
- CTLA4: cytotoxic T-lymphocyte–associated antigen 4
- DHFR: dihydrofolate reductase
- DOE: dyspnea on exertion
- DPD: dihydropyrimidine dehydrogenase
- DVT: deep vein thrombosis
- EF: ejection fraction
- EGFR: epidermal growth factor receptor
- EKG: electrocardiogram
- ERK2: extracellular signal–related kinase 2
- Fc: fragment crystallizable
- FGFR: fibroblast growth factor receptor
- FKBP-12: FK506-binding protein-12
- FLT3: FMS-related tyrosine kinase receptor-3
- FOLFIRI: folinic acid/fluorouracil/irinotecan
- FOLR1: folate receptor 1
- FPGS: folylpolyglutamate synthetase
- GARFT: glycinamide ribonucleotide formyltransferase
- GE: gastroesophageal
- GERD: gastroesophageal reflux disease
- GGT: γ-glutamyl transferase
- GI: gastrointestinal
- GM-CSF: granulocyte-macrophage colony-stimulating factor
- HCC: hepatocellular carcinoma

- HDAC: histone deacetylase
- HER2: human epidermal growth factor receptor 2
- HSV: herpes simplex virus
- IDH: isocitrate dehydrogenase
- Ig: immunoglobulin
- IGF-1R: insulin-like growth factor-1 receptor
- ITD: internal tandem duplication
- ITP: immune thrombocytopenic purpura
- JAK: Janus kinase
- KDR: kinase insert domain receptor
- KLF4: Kruppel-like factor 4
- KRAS: Kirsten rat sarcoma
- LD: lactate dehydrogenase
- LVEF: left ventricular ejection fraction
- mAb: monoclonal antibody
- MAPK: mitogen-activated protein kinase
- MCL: mantle cell lymphoma
- mCRC: metastatic colorectal cancer
- MDS: myelodysplastic syndrome
- MEK1: mitogen-activated protein kinase kinase 1
- MET: mesenchymal–epithelial transition
- MM: multiple myeloma
- MTC: medullary thyroid carcinoma
- MTF-1: metal-regulatory transcription factor 1
- mTOR: mammalian target of rapamycin

- MWF: Monday, Wednesday, Friday
- NHL: non-Hodgkin lymphoma
- NRAS: neuroblastoma RAS viral oncogene homolog
- NSCLC: non–small-cell lung cancer
- NTRK: neurotrophic tropomyosin receptor kinase
- PAP: prostatic-acid phosphatase
- PARP: poly (ADP-ribose) polymerase
- PDGFR: platelet-derived growth factor receptor
- PD-L1: programmed death ligand 1
- PEG: polyethylene glycol
- PFS: progression-free survival
- PI3K: phosphatidylinositol 3-kinase
- PIP3: phosphatidylinositol-3,4,5-trisphosphate
- PKC: protein kinase C
- pNET: pancreatic neuroendocrine tumor
- PTCH: patched
- PTCL: peripheral T-cell lymphoma
- RANKL: receptor activator of nuclear factor-κB ligand
- RAS: rat sarcoma virus
- RET: rearranged during transfection
- RFC-1: reduced folate carrier
- RTKs: receptor tyrosine kinases
- SAPK: stress-activated protein kinase
- SCCHN: squamous cell carcinoma of the head and neck
- scFv: single-chain variable fragment

- SCLC: small-cell lung cancer
- SMO: small-molecule smoothened
- STAT3: signal transducer and activator of transcription 3
- STS: soft-tissue sarcoma
- SYK: spleen tyrosine kinase
- TAA: tumor-associated antigen
- TCR: T-cell receptor
- TEN: toxic epidermal necrolysis
- TGF: transforming growth factor
- TLS: tumor lysis syndrome
- TRK: tropomyosin receptor kinase
- TS: thymidylate synthase
- URI: upper respiratory infection
- VEGF: vascular endothelial growth factor
- VEGFR: vascular endothelial growth factor receptor
- XRT: radiotherapy

Abemaciclib

- **Alias:** LY2835219
- **Brand Name:** Verzenio
- **Type Mechanism:** CDK4/6 inhibitor blocks early G1 retinoblastoma (Rb) protein phosphorylation and G1-S cell-cycle transition.
- **Drug Class:** Cyclin-dependent kinase inhibitor
- **Mechanism of Action:** CDK4/6 inhibitor
- **FDA Approval Date:** September 28, 2017
- **Indications:** Advanced or metastatic breast cancer with hormone receptor (HR) (+) and HER2(−) in combination with aromatase inhibitors as an initial endocrine-based therapy or in combination with fulvestrant with disease progression following prior endocrine therapy; as monotherapy for the treatment of adult patients with HR-positive, HER2-negative advanced or MBC with disease progression following endocrine therapy and prior chemotherapy in the metastatic setting; in combination with endocrine therapy (tamoxifen or an aromatase inhibitor) for the adjuvant treatment of adult patients with HR-positive, HER2-negative, node-positive, early breast cancer at high risk of recurrence and a Ki-67 score ≥20% as determined by an FDA-approved test

- **Dose:** 150 to 200 mg twice daily (BID)
- **Half-life:** 18.3 hours
- **Metabolism:** Major CYP3A4 substrate
- **Side Effects:** Diarrhea, neutropenia and leukopenia, nausea, abdominal pain, infections, fatigue, anemia, alopecia, decreased appetite, vomiting, transaminitis, headache
- **Clinical Pearls:** Need premedication with 5HT3 antagonist before each dose. Considered as moderate-to-high emetogenic potential.

Abiraterone Acetate

- **Alias:** CB7630
- **Brand Name:** Zytiga; Yonsa (micronized formulation)
- **Type Mechanism:** Selectively and irreversibly inhibits 17-α-hydroxylase/C17,20-lyase (CYP17), an enzyme required for testosterone synthesis. The inhibition of CYP17 results in increased mineralocorticoid production by the adrenals and suppression of testosterone production by both the testes and the adrenals.
- **Drug Class:** Androgen inhibitor
- **Mechanism of Action:** CYP17 inhibitor
- **FDA Approval Date:** April 28, 2011

- **Indications:** 2011 approved for late-stage prostate cancer; 2018 approval for the treatment of earlier form of metastatic prostate cancer with prednisone
- **Dose:** 1,000 mg orally (PO) daily with prednisone. Give on a fasting stomach 1 hour before and 2 hours after meal.
- **Half-life:** 14.4 to 16.5 hours
- **Metabolism:** Major CYP3A4 substrate
- **Side Effects:** Peripheral edema, fatigue, hypertension (HTN), hyperglycemia/hypertriglyceridemia, lymphopenia, transaminitis, arthralgias/myalgias, diarrhea
- **Clinical Pearls:** Yonza™ (micronized formulation) may be taken regardless of meals; patient should also be receiving gonadotropin-releasing hormone (GnRH) analog concurrently or have had a bilateral orchiectomy.

Acalisib

- **Alias:** GS-9820
- **Type Mechanism:** A second-generation inhibitor of the β and δ isoforms of the 110-kDa catalytic subunit of class IA PI3K that inhibits the activity of PI3K, thereby preventing the production of the second messenger PIP3, which decreases tumor cell proliferation and induces cell death
- **Drug Class:** PI3K inhibitor
- **Phase:** Phase 1/2
- **Indications:** Relapsed/refractory lymphoid malignancies (CLL and B-cell lymphomas)
- **Dose:** 200 to 400 mg PO BID
- **Side Effects:** Diarrhea, rash, weight loss, ALT/AST elevations, dysgeusia, fever, nausea, neutropenia, anemia, increased SCr, pneumonia

(Kater et al., 2018)

Adavosertib

- **Alias:** AZD1775; MK-1775
- **Type Mechanism:** It selectively targets and inhibits WEE1, a tyrosine kinase that phosphorylates cyclin-dependent kinase 1 (CDK1, CDC2) to inactivate the CDC2/cyclin B complex. Inhibition of WEE1 activity prevents the phosphorylation of CDC2 and impairs the G2 DNA damage checkpoint.
- **Drug Class:** Cell-cycle inhibitor
- **Mechanism of Action:** WEE1 inhibitor
- **Phase:** Phase 2
- **Indications:** Phase 2 combination with olaparib in recurrent ovarian, primary peritoneal, or fallopian tube cancer; phase 2 studies in advanced solid tumors that have SETD2 mutation; phase 2 in recurrent uterine serous carcinoma or uterine carcinosarcoma

- **Dose:** Intermittent dosing daily to BID for 5 days on, 2 days off, or Q other week 5 days on, 2 days off with dose ranging from 200 to 300 mg on empty stomach with or without chemotherapy/biotherapy
- **Half-life:** 18.3 hours
- **Metabolism:** Major substrate of CYP3A4
- **Side Effects:** Nausea, vomiting—can be controlled by using 5HT3 + steroids as premedications; fatigue, diarrhea, anemia, thrombocytopenia, and leukopenia/neutropenia; loss of appetite
- **Clinical Pearls:** High-fat meal was shown not to have clinically relevant effect on exposure of adavosertib, suggesting that it can be dosed regardless of meals.

(Kato et al., 2020; Nagard et al., 2020)

Ado-Trastuzumab Emtansine

- **Alias:** T-DM1; trastuzumab-DM1; trastuzumab-MCC-DM1
- **Brand Name:** Kadcyla
- **Type Mechanism:** A HER2 antibody–drug conjugate (ADC) that incorporates the HER2-targeted actions of trastuzumab with the microtubule inhibitor DM1 (a maitansine derivative). The conjugate, which is linked via a stable thioether linker, allows for selective delivery into HER2 overexpressing cells, resulting in cell-cycle arrest and apoptosis.

- **Drug Class:** ADC
- **Mechanism of Action:** HER2 ADC
- **FDA Approval Date:** February 22, 2013
- **Indications:** HER2-positive metastatic breast cancer patients who have previously had trastuzumab-based treatment with taxanes; the adjuvant treatment of patients with HER2-positive early breast cancer who have residual invasive disease after neoadjuvant taxane and trastuzumab-based treatment
- **Dose:** 3.6 mg/kg intravenous (IV) Q 3 weeks over 90 minutes with the first dose, then may decrease to 30 minutes if tolerated
- **Half-life:** 4 days
- **Metabolism:** Major CYP3A4 substrate
- **Side Effects:** Fatigue, headache, neuropathy, skin rash, nausea, stomatitis, abdominal pain, muscle pain, arthralgias, cough, fever, thrombocytopenia, anemia

Afatinib Dimaleate

- **Brand Name:** Gilotrif
- **Type Mechanism:** A dimaleate salt form of afatinib, an orally bioavailable anilinoquinazoline derivative and inhibitor of the RTK EGFR (ErbB). Upon administration, afatinib selectively and irreversibly binds to and inhibits the epidermal growth factor receptors

1 (ErbB1; EGFR), 2 (ErbB2; HER2), and 4 (ErbB4; HER4), and certain EGFR mutants, including those caused by EGFR exon 19 deletion mutations or exon 21 (L858R) mutations. In addition, afatinib inhibits the EGFR T790M gatekeeper mutation, which is resistant to the treatment with the first-generation EGFR inhibitors. EGFR, HER2, and HER4 are RTKs that belong to the EGFR superfamily.

- **Drug Class:** EGFR inhibitor
- **Mechanism of Action:** A TKI that covalently binds to EGFR (ErbB1), HER2 (ErbB2), and HER4 (ErbB4) to irreversibly inhibit tyrosine kinase autophosphorylation and downregulate ErbB signaling
- **FDA Approval Date:** July 12, 2013
- **Indications:** Metastatic EGFR mutation–positive NSCLC and metastatic squamous cell lung cancer
- **Dose:** 40 mg PO daily. Administer ≥1 hour before or 2 hours after a meal.
- **Half-life:** 37 hours
- **Metabolism:** P-glycoprotein/ABCB1 major substrate
- **Side Effects:** Acneiform eruption, skin rash, paronychia, xeroderma, pruritis, cheilitis, diarrhea, stomatitis, nausea, vomiting, lymphocytopenia, transaminitis, hyperbilirubinemia, hypokalemia
- **Clinical Pearls:** Binding to T790M can lead to longer time to resistance.

Afuresertib

- **Alias:** GSK2110183
- **Type Mechanism:** Inhibitor of the serine/threonine protein kinase Akt (protein kinase B) with potential antineoplastic activity. Afuresertib binds to and inhibits the activity of Akt, which may result in inhibition of the PI3K/Akt signaling pathway and tumor cell proliferation and the induction of tumor cell apoptosis.
- **Drug Class:** AKT inhibitor
- **Mechanism of Action:** Inhibitor of protein kinase B (AKT)/PI3K pathway
- **Phase:** Phase 1/2
- **Indications:** Undergoing trials in platinum-resistant ovarian cancer, MCRPC, and relapsed/refractory MM
- **Dose:** 125 mg PO daily in combination with paclitaxel and carboplatin
- **Half-life:** 1.7 days
- **Side Effects:** Nausea, diarrhea, dyspepsia, fatigue, gastrointestinal (GI) reflux, rash, neutropenia, odynophagia, asthenia
- **Clinical Pearls:** Most useful in tumors with PTEN deficiency and PIK3 mutations

(Nitulescu et al., 2016; Spencer et al., 2014)

Alisertib

- **Alias:** MLN8237
- **Type Mechanism:** Second-generation, orally bioavailable, selective binding to and inhibiting Aurora A kinase in cells. Inhibition of Aurora A results in delayed mitotic entry and progression through mitosis, leading to an accumulation of cells with a tetraploid DNA content. This results in a process called *mitotic slippage*, causing apoptosis, senescence, or reenter the cell cycle.
- **Drug Class:** Mitotic inhibitor
- **Mechanism of Action:** Aurora kinase inhibitor
- **Phase:** Phase 2/3
- **Indications:** Phase 2 in relapsed/refractory neuroblastoma; phase 3 relapsed/refractory PTCL; phase 2 SCLC, CRPC, and neuroendocrine prostate cancer; phase 2 high-risk AML
- **Dose:** 50 mg BID for 7 consecutive days of the 21-day cycle (10 mg enteric coated tablet). Fast 2 hours before and 1 hour after dosing
- **Half-life:** 19 to 23 hours
- **Metabolism:** Excreted primarily unchanged
- **Side Effects:** Fatigue, neutropenia, nausea, stomatitis, HTN

(DuBois et al., 2018; O'Connor et al., 2019)

Alpelisib

- **Alias:** BYL719
- **Brand Name:** Piqray
- **Type Mechanism:** An orally bioavailable PI3K inhibitor that specifically inhibits PIK3 in the PI3K/AKT kinase (or protein kinase B) signaling pathway, thereby inhibiting the activation of the PI3K signaling pathway. This may result in inhibition of tumor cell growth and survival in susceptible tumor cell populations; inhibits the PI3K-α isoform and much less strongly the β, δ, and γ isoforms.
- **Mechanism of Action:** PI3 kinase inhibitor
- **FDA Approval Date:** May 24, 2019
- **Indications:** Breast cancer, advanced or metastatic (HR positive, HER2 negative, PIK3CA mutated)
- **Dose:** 300 mg PO once daily
- **Half-life:** 8 to 9 hours
- **Metabolism:** Minor CYP3A4 substrate; BCRP/ABCG2 substrate
- **Side Effects:** Hyperglycemia, erythematous rash, xeroderma, edema, stomatitis, nausea/vomiting, diarrhea, fatigue, anorexia, increased lipase, lymphopenia, thrombocytopenia, prolonged partial thromboplastin time (PTT), elevated ALT, increased SCr

Alrizomadlin

- **Alias:** APG 115
- **Type Mechanism:** Activates the p53/p21 pathway to restore p53 function by inhibiting the MDM2, a mouse double minute 2 homolog. This results in potent antiproliferative and apoptogenic activities and induces cell-cycle arrest in p53 wild type (WT).
- **Drug Class:** MDM2 antagonist
- **Phase:** Phase 2
- **Indications:** p53 WT salivary gland carcinoma, relapsed/refractory unresectable or metastatic melanoma, NSCLC, malignant peripheral nerve sheath tumor, liposarcoma, ATM-mutant solid tumors, and urothelial carcinoma
- **Dose:** 100 mg PO every other day (QOD) for 2 weeks on, 1 week off (in combination with pembrolizumab)
- **Side Effects:** Nausea, thrombocytopenia, vomiting, fatigue, loss of appetite, diarrhea, neutropenia, pain in extremity, anemia
- **Clinical Pearls:** It has been granted a fast track designation by the FDA for the treatment of relapsed/refractory unresectable or metastatic melanoma who are relapsed or refractory to prior immune-oncologic agents.

(Rasco et al., 2019)

Altiratinib

- **Alias:** DC-2701; DP-5164
- **Type Mechanism:** Inhibitor of c-Met/ hepatocyte growth factor receptor (HGFR), VEGFR2, Tie2 RTK (TIE2), and TRK
- **Drug Class:** Multitargeted TKI
- **Mechanism of Action:** MET/TIE2/VEFGR2/ TRK (A, B, C) kinase inhibitor
- **Phase:** Phase 1
- **Indications:** Solid tumors
- **Dose:** PO BID for a 28-day cycle

AMG337

- **Type Mechanism:** A small molecule that inhibits the enzymatic activity of the c-Met tyrosine kinase
- **Drug Class:** c-MET inhibitor
- **Mechanism of Action:** c-Met inhibitor selectively binds to c-Met, thereby disrupting c-Met signal transduction pathways. This may induce cell death in tumor cells overexpressing c-Met protein or expressing constitutively activated c-Met protein.
- **Phase:** Phase 2
- **Indications:** MET-amplified GE junction (GEJ) cancer, gastric cancer, and esophageal cancer

- **Dose:** RP2D: 300 mg PO daily
- **Half-life:** 5.9 to 7 hours
- **Side Effects:** Headache, nausea/vomiting, fatigue, constipation, abdominal pain, peripheral edema, rash

(Kwak et al., 2015)

Anastrozole

- **Alias:** ICI-D1033; ZD1033
- **Brand Name:** Arimidex
- **Type Mechanism:** A potent and selective nonsteroidal aromatase inhibitor. By inhibiting aromatase, the conversion of androstenedione to estrone, and testosterone to estradiol, is prevented, thereby decreasing tumor mass or delaying progression in patients with tumors responsive to hormones. Anastrozole can cause an 85% decrease in estrone sulfate levels.
- **Drug Class:** Aromatase inhibitor
- **Mechanism of Action:** A potent and selective nonsteroidal aromatase inhibitor
- **FDA Approval Date:** December 27, 1995
- **Indications:** HR-positive breast cancer; off-label endometrial and uterine carcinoma; off-label recurrent ovarian cancer
- **Dose:** 1 mg PO daily regardless of meals
- **Half-life:** ~50 hours

- **Side Effects:** Hot flash, nausea, GI distress, skin rash, depression, fatigue, headache, mood disorder, pharyngitis, arthralgia, arthritis, hypercholesterolemia, transaminitis, osteoporosis

Andecaliximab (GS-5745)

- **Alias:** GS-5745
- **Type Mechanism:** A mAb that inhibits matrix metalloproteinase 9 (MMP9), an extracellular enzyme involved in matrix remodeling, tumor growth, and metastasis. Increased MMP9 expression is associated with poor prognosis across many malignancies, including gastric cancer.
- **Drug Class:** MMP9 mAb inhibitor
- **Mechanism of Action:** A mAb inhibitor of the MMP9
- **Phase:** Phase 2
- **Indications:** Advanced pancreatic adenocarcinoma, NSCLC, HER2 (−) GEJ adenocarcinoma, and gastric cancer
- **Dose:** 800 mg IV on days 1 and 15 of the 28-day cycle
- **Half-life:** 2.4 to 8.3 days
- **Side Effects:** Neutropenia, diarrhea, fatigue, nausea

(Shah et al., 2018)

Anetumab Ravtansine

- **Alias:** BAY94-9343
- **Type Mechanism:** An ADC that is a fully human anti-mesothelin antibody (MF-T) coupled via a reducible disulfide linker to a microtubule-targeting toxophore DM4, binds to mesothelin with high affinity and delivers the microtubule inhibitor DM4 to mesothelin-positive tumor cells
- **Drug Class:** ADC
- **Mechanism of Action:** Anti-mesothelin ADC
- **Phase:** Phase 2 in mesothelin-expressing solid tumors
- **Indications:** Ovarian cancer, pancreatic cancer, NSCLC; indication for mesothelioma did not meet PFS—clinical trial stopped in July 2017 for mesothelioma
- **Dose:** 6.5 mg/kg IV once Q 3 weeks; 1.8 to 2.2 mg/kg IV Q week
- **Half-life:** 4 to 5 days
- **Side Effects:** Fatigue, weakness, neuropathy, nausea, vomiting, anorexia, keratitis/keratopathy

(Chokshi & Hochster, 2018)

Anlotinib

- **Alias:** ALTN HCl
- **Type Mechanism:** Targets multiple RTKs, including VEGFR2 and VEGFR3
- **Drug Class:** VEGF inhibitor
- **Mechanism of Action:** Receptor TKI of VEGFR2/3; can also inhibit both tumor angiogenesis and tumor cell proliferation.
- **Phase:** Phase 3
- **Indications:** Alveolar soft-part sarcoma, leiomyosarcoma, synovial sarcoma
- **Dose:** 12 mg PO daily for 14 days on, 7 days off
- **Half-life:** 116 hours
- **Side Effects:** HTN, fatigue, thyroid-stimulating hormone (TSH) elevation, anorexia, hypertriglyceridemia, hand-foot syndrome, hypercholesterolemia, GGT elevation

(Han et al., 2018; Shen et al., 2018)

Apalutamide

- **Alias:** ARN-509; JNJ-56021927
- **Brand Name:** Erleada
- **Type Mechanism:** Binds directly to the AR ligand-binding domain to prevent AR translocation, DNA binding, and receptor-mediated transcription. AR inhibition results in decreased proliferation of tumor cells and increased apoptosis, leading to a decrease in tumor volume.
- **Drug Class:** A nonsteroidal AR inhibitor

- **Mechanism of Action:** AR inhibitor
- **FDA Approval Date:** February 14, 2018
- **Indications:** Metastatic castrate-sensitive prostate cancer; nonmetastatic castrate-resistant prostate cancer (MCRPC)
- **Dose:** 240 mg PO daily (in combination with androgen deprivation therapy)
- **Half-life:** ~3 days
- **Metabolism:** Major CYP2C8 substrate; potent inducer of CYP2C19, CYP3A4, and P-glycoprotein
- **Side Effects:** HTN, peripheral edema, rash, pruritus, hot flash, hypercholesterolemia, hyperglycemia, hypertriglyceridemia, nausea, anemia, lymphopenia, fatigue, arthralgia

Apatinib

- **Alias:** YN968D1; rivoceranib (international nonproprietary name)
- **Type Mechanism:** Orally bioavailable VEGFR2 (KDR) inhibitor; also mildly inhibits RET, KIT, and SRC
- **Drug Class:** Antiangiogenic TKI
- **Mechanism of Action:** Selectively inhibits VEGFR2
- **Phase:** Phase 3 gastric cancer and HCC; FDA granted orphan status in adenoid cystic carcinoma; phase 2 in CRC

- **FDA Approval Date:** Orphan status for adenoid cystic carcinoma
- **Indications:** Gastric cancer, CRC, adenoid cystic carcinoma, HCC
- **Dose:** 850 mg daily in 2 divided doses; optimum dose seen is 500 mg daily.
- **Half-life:** 9 hours
- **Metabolism:** Extensively by CYP3A4/5
- **Side Effects:** HTN, hand-foot syndrome, diarrhea, anemia, thrombocytopenia, neutropenia, proteinuria, fatigue
- **Clinical Pearls:** UGT1A4 and UT2B7 deficiency may affect metabolism of apatinib.

(Du et al., 2020)

Atezolizumab

- **Alias:** MPDL3280A; RO5541267
- **Brand Name:** Tecentriq
- **Type Mechanism:** A humanized mAb inhibiting PD-L1
- **Drug Class:** A humanized mAb immune checkpoint inhibitor
- **Mechanism of Action:** Binds to PD-L1 to selectively prevent the interaction between the programmed cell death-1 (PD-1) and B7.1. PD-L1 is an immune checkpoint protein expressed on tumor cells and tumor-infiltrating cells and downregulates

antitumor T-cell function by binding to PD-1 and B7.1; blocking PD-1 and B7.1 interactions restores antitumor T-cell function.

- **FDA Approval Date:** May 18, 2016 For breast cancer, March 8, 2019 Voluntary withdrawal (Roche), September 25, 2021. Approval remains active for other tumor types.
- **Indications:** PD-L1–positive triple-negative breast cancer (SP142 assay); urothelial cancer ineligible for platinum-containing chemotherapy; metastatic NSCLC; SCLC; metastatic HCC; metastatic melanoma
- **Dose:** 840 mg IV Q 2 weeks; 1,200 mg IV Q 3 weeks; or 1,680 mg IV Q 4 weeks
- **Half-life:** 27 days
- **Side Effects:** Peripheral edema, fatigue, skin rash, hyponatremia, decreased appetite, transaminitis, hyperbilirubinemia, infection
- **Clinical Pearls:** When combining with chemotherapy, administer atezolizumab first

Avapritinib

- **Alias:** BLU-285
- **Brand Name:** Ayvakit™
- **Type Mechanism:** A potent TKI that blocks PDGFRα
- **Drug Class:** PDGFRα TKI
- **Mechanism of Action:** Targets PDGFRα and PDGFR D842 mutants, as well as KIT exon 11, 11/17, and 17 mutants. It also inhibits autophosphorylation of KIT D816V and PDGFRα D842V, which are mutants associated with resistance to approved kinase inhibitors.
- **FDA Approval Date:** January 9, 2020
- **Indications:** Metastatic gastrointestinal stromal tumor (GIST) with a PDGFRα exon 18 mutation
- **Dose:** 300 mg PO daily
- **Half-life:** 32 to 57 hours
- **Metabolism:** Major CYP3A4 substrate
- **Side Effects:** Edema, hair discoloration, skin rash, dyspepsia, decreased serum albumin, constipation, decreased appetite, diarrhea, neutropenia, transaminitis, cognitive dysfunction, dizziness, fatigue, headache, sleep disorder
- **Clinical Pearls:** Need antiemetics owing to moderate or high emetogenicity

Avelumab

- **Alias:** MSB0010718C
- **Brand Name:** Bavencio
- **Type Mechanism:** Fully human mAb that binds to PD-L1 to selectively prevent the interaction between PD-1 and 7.1 receptors,

resulting in the restoration of antitumor T-cell function

- **Drug Class:** Anti-PD-L1 mAb
- **FDA Approval Date:** March 23, 2017
- **Indications:** Metastatic Merkel cell carcinoma; locally, advanced, or metastatic urothelial carcinoma following platinum therapy; advanced renal cell carcinoma (RCC)
- **Dose:** 10 mg/kg IV over 60 minutes Q 2 weeks (for gestational trophoblastic neoplasia chemotherapy resistant) or 800 mg (FLAT dose) IV Q 2 weeks; should premedicate with acetaminophen and diphenhydramine for the first four infusions
- **Half-life:** 6.1 days
- **Side Effects:** Peripheral edema, HTN, fatigue, dizziness, skin rash, nausea, diarrhea, hyponatremia, decreased appetite, abdominal pain, transaminitis, arthralgia, infusion-related reaction with chills, fevers

Axitinib

- **Alias:** AG-013736
- **Brand Name:** Inlyta
- **Type Mechanism:** Selective second-generation, orally bioavailable inhibitor of VEGFRs (VEGFR1, VEGFR2, and VEGFR3), PDGFR, and KIT

- **Drug Class:** VEGF TKI
- **FDA Approval Date:** January 27, 2012
- **Indications:** Advanced RCC; off-label use for differentiated thyroid cancer
- **Dose:** Optimum dose is 10 mg PO BID; recommend to dose escalate Q 2 weeks starting at 5 mg.
- **Half-life:** 2 to 6 hours
- **Metabolism:** Major CYP3A4 substrate and UGT1A1 substrate
- **Side Effects:** Diarrhea, HTN, fatigue, decreased appetite, palmar–plantar erythrodysesthesia, skin rash, stomatitis, hypothyroidism, transaminitis, increased SCr, nausea/vomiting
- **Clinical Pearls:** Dysphonia (hoarseness) may occur while taking. Advise patients to avoid irritants and to drink plenty of fluids.

Belinostat

- **Alias:** PXD101
- **Brand Name:** Beleodaq
- **Type Mechanism:** A novel hydroxamic acid–type HDAC inhibitor that targets HDAC enzymes, thereby inhibiting tumor cell proliferation, inducing apoptosis, promoting cellular differentiation, and inhibiting angiogenesis

- **Drug Class:** HDAC inhibitor
- **Mechanism of Action:** An HDAC inhibitor that catalyzes acetyl group removal from protein lysine residues (of histone and some nonhistone proteins). Inhibition of HDAC results in accumulation of acetyl groups, leading to cell-cycle arrest and apoptosis. Belinostat has preferential cytotoxicity toward tumor cells versus normal cells.
- **FDA Approval Date:** July 3, 2014
- **Indications:** Relapsed/refractory PTCL
- **Dose:** 1,000 mg/m^2 IV on days 1 to 5 Q 21 days
- **Half-life:** 1.1 hours
- **Metabolism:** Weak substrates of CYP2C9, CYP3A4, P-glycoprotein/ABCB1, and UGT1A1
- **Side Effects:** Peripheral edema, prolonged QT, fatigue, chills, headache, rash, pruritus, hypokalemia, anemia, thrombocytopenia, dyspnea, fevers, hypotension, elevated SCr
- **Clinical Pearls:** Dose only if absolute neutrophil count (ANC) is ≥1,000/mm^3 and platelets ≥50,000/mm^3. NOTE: If the patient is homozygous for UGT1A1*28 allele, reduce the initial dose to 750 mg/m^2.

Bemarituzumab

- **Alias:** FPA144
- **Type Mechanism:** A glycoengineered, humanized mAb directed against the FGFR2b that specifically binds to and inhibits FGFR2b on tumor cell surfaces, which prevents FGFR2 from binding to its ligands, FGFR2b activation, and the activation of FGFR2b-mediated signal transduction pathways. The binding of bemarituzumab to FGFR2b protein also induces ADCC against FGFR2b-expressing tumor cells.
- **Phase:** Phase 2/3
- **Indications:** GE adenocarcinoma or gastric carcinoma with FGFR2b overexpression
- **Dose:** 15 mg/kg IV Q 2 weeks in combination with mFOLFOX
- **Half-life:** 12.8 days
- **Side Effects:** Fatigue, nausea, dry eyes, anemia, neutropenia, increased AST, vomiting, infusion reaction

(Catenacci et al., 2020)

Bempegaldesleukin

- **Type Mechanism:** A PEGylated interleukin-2 (IL-2) acting as a CD122-preferential IL-2

pathway agonist designed to activate and proliferate CD8$^+$ T cells and NK cells
- **Phase:** Phase 3
- **Indications:** Metastatic melanoma
- **Dose:** 0.006 mg/kg IV Q 3 weeks
- **Half-life:** 20 hours
- **Side Effects:** Flulike symptoms, rash, fatigue, hypotension

(Khushalani et al., 2020)

Berzosertib

- **Alias:** VX-970; M6620
- **Type Mechanism:** An inhibitor of ataxia telangiectasia and rad3-related (ATR) kinase, a DNA damage response kinase that selectively binds to and inhibits ATR kinase activity and prevents ATR-mediated signaling in the ATR-checkpoint kinase 1 (CHK1) signaling pathway. This prevents DNA damage checkpoint activation, disrupts DNA damage repair, and induces tumor cell apoptosis.
- **Drug Class:** ATR inhibitor
- **Phase:** Phase 2
- **Indications:** mCRC, small-cell neuroendocrine cancers, platinum-resistant SCLC, and platinum-resistant serous ovarian cancer harboring molecular aberrations, including ATM loss and an ARID1A mutation

- **Dose:** 240 mg/m^2 IV once weekly or twice weekly as monotherapy or 90 mg/m^2 IV weekly (combined with carboplatin AUC5)
- **Half-life:** 18.5 hours for once weekly dosing; 12.8 hours for twice weekly dosing; 14.3 hours for combination therapy
- **Side Effects:** Flushing, nausea, pruritus, headache, infusion-related side effects, such as flushing, fatigue, thrombocytopenia, neutropenia, and anemia

(Yap et al., 2020)

Bevacizumab

- **Brand Name:** Avastin
- **Type Mechanism:** A recombinant humanized mAb directed against the VEGF, a proangiogenic cytokine
  - Binds to VEGF and inhibits receptor binding, thereby preventing the growth and maintenance of tumor blood vessels
- **Drug Class:** VEGF inhibitor
- **FDA Approval Date:** February 26, 2004
- **Indications:** Colon, lung, and renal carcinomas and glioblastoma multiforme
- **Dose:** 5 to 10 mg/kg IV Q 2 weeks or 15 mg/kg IV Q 3 weeks
- **Half-life:** 20 days

- **Side Effects:** HTN, severe or fatal hemorrhage (GI bleed, hemoptysis, central nervous system [CNS] bleed), bowel perforation, fistulas/abscess formation, proteinuria
- **Clinical Pearls:** Have patients monitor blood pressure and bring the log to appointments. Avoid use in patients with severe hypertension requiring multiple antihypertensive medications for control.

BI 811283

- **Type Mechanism:** Binds to and inhibits Aurora kinases, resulting in disruption of the assembly of the mitotic spindle apparatus, disruption of chromosome segregation, and inhibition of cell proliferation
- **Drug Class:** AURKB inhibitor
- **Mechanism of Action:** A small-molecule inhibitor of the serine/threonine protein kinase Aurora kinase
- **Phase:** Phase 1
- **Dose:** 230 mg as 24-hour continuous infusion on day 1 of a 21-day cycle
- **Half-life:** 12 to 26 hours
- **Side Effects:** Neutropenia, leukopenia, febrile neutropenia, fatigue, alopecia, diarrhea, decreased appetite

(Mross et al., 2016)

Bicalutamide

- **Alias:** CDX; ICI-176334
- **Brand Name:** Casodex
- **Type Mechanism:** A pure nonsteroidal AR inhibitor, specifically a competitive inhibitor for the binding of dihydrotestosterone and testosterone
- **Drug Class:** Antiandrogen
- **FDA Approval Date:** October 4, 1995
- **Indications:** Metastatic prostate cancer
- **Dose:** 50 mg PO daily
- **Half-life:** 6 days
- **Metabolism:** Substrate of CYP3A4
- **Side Effects:** AST and ALT increase, hyperbilirubinemia, ALP increase, nausea, pain (bone, back, pelvis), anorexia, fatigue, diarrhea, hot flashes, limb edema
- **Clinical Pearls:** Use in combination with luteinizing hormone–releasing hormone (LHRH) analog such as leuprolide.

Binimetinib

- **Alias:** ARRY-162; MEK162; ARRY-43162
- **Type Mechanism:** An orally available inhibitor of MEK1/2 prevents the activation of MEK1/2-dependent effector proteins and transcription factors, which may result in the inhibition of growth factor–mediated cell signaling. This may eventually lead to

an inhibition of tumor cell proliferation and an inhibition in the production of various inflammatory cytokines, including IL-1, IL-6, and tumor necrosis factor (TNF).

- **Drug Class:** MEK1/2 inhibitor
- **FDA Approval Date:** June 27, 2018
- **Indications:** Unresectable or metastatic melanoma; off-label use for metastatic, refractory, RAS WT, and BRAF V600E–mutant CRC
- **Dose:** 45 mg PO Q 12 hours
- **Half-life:** 3.5 hours
- **Metabolism:** BCRP/ABCG2 substrate; UGT1A1 substrate
- **Side Effects:** Skin rash, fatigue, dermatitis acneiform, peripheral edema, diarrhea, nausea, elevated CPK, anemia, increased GGT, transaminitis
- **Clinical Pearls:** Use in combination with encorafenib in melanoma.

Bintrafusp Alfa

- **Alias:** M7824; MSB0011359C
- **Type Mechanism:** A first-in-class bifunctional fusion protein composed of the extracellular domain of TGF-β receptor 2 (a TGF-β "trap") fused to a human IgG1 antibody blocking PD-L1
- **Drug Class:** TGF-β/PD-L1 inhibitor
- **Phase:** Phase 1/2

- **Indications:** NSCLC; biliary tract cancer including ampullary cancer, intrahepatic and extrahepatic cholangiocarcinoma
- **Dose:** RP2D: 1,200 mg IV Q 2 weeks
- **Side Effects:** Rash, fever, maculopapular rash, increased lipase, pruritis

(Vugmeyster et al., 2020)

BMS-936559

- **Alias:** MDX1105
- **Type Mechanism:** High-affinity, fully humanized PD-L1–specific IgG4 mAb that inhibits the binding of PD-L1 to both PD-1 and CD80
- **Phase:** No active clinical trials for cancer in the United States; previous studies in melanoma and hematologic malignancies were withdrawn.
- **Indications:** Advanced solid tumors, especially melanoma, RCC, NSCLC, and ovarian cancer
- **Dose:** 0.3 to 10 mg/kg as 60-minute infusion Q 2 weeks
- **Half-life:** 15 days
- **Side Effects:** Rash, pruritis, hypothyroidism related to hypophysitis, hepatitis, diarrhea
- **Clinical Pearls:** May require antihistamines and antipyretics as premedications

(Brahmer et al., 2012; Gay et al., 2017)

Brigatinib

- **Alias:** AP26113
- **Brand Name:** Alunbrig
- **Type Mechanism:** A broad-spectrum multikinase inhibitor with activity against ALK, ROS1, IGF-1R, and FLT3, as well as EGFR deletion and point mutations. ALK autophosphorylation and ALK-mediated phosphorylation of downstream signaling proteins STAT3, AKT, ERK1/2, and S6 are inhibited by brigatinib.
- **Mechanism of Action:** ALK and EGFR kinase inhibitor. ALK is a member of the insulin receptor superfamily.
- **FDA Approval Date:** April 28, 2017
- **Indications:** ALK(+), metastatic NSCLC
- **Dose:** 90 mg PO daily for 7 days. If tolerated, may continue to full dose at 180 mg PO daily
- **Half-life:** 25 hours
- **Metabolism:** Major CYP3A4 substrate; BCRP/ABCG2 substrate
- **Side Effects:** HTN, fatigue, headache, peripheral neuropathy, skin rash including palmar–plantar erythrodysesthesia, hyperglycemia, transaminitis, constipation or diarrhea, nausea, anemia, lymphocytopenia, cough, prolonged PTT, neutropenia, bradycardia, angioedema, pruritus

Buparlisib

- **Alias:** BKM120
- **Type Mechanism:** Inhibits class I PIK3 in the PI3K/AKT kinase (or protein kinase B) signaling pathway in an adenosine triphosphate (ATP)-competitive manner, thereby inhibiting the production of the secondary messenger PIP3 and activation of the PI3K signaling pathway. This may result in inhibition of tumor cell growth and survival in susceptible tumor cell populations.
- **Mechanism of Action:** Pan-PI3K inhibitor
- **Phase:** Phase 2/3
- **Indications:** HER2—advanced, metastatic breast cancer; platinum-pretreated recurrent or metastatic SCCHN
- **Dose:** 100 mg PO daily in combination with fulvestrant. Take dose 1 hour after breakfast and fast for 2 hours after dosing.
- **Half-life:** 40 hours
- **Metabolism:** Moderate/reversible inhibitor of CYP3A4
- **Side Effects:** Rash, anorexia, mood alteration, diarrhea, hyperglycemia, elevated ALT, fatigue, pyrexia, pneumonitis
- **Clinical Pearls:** Studies in advanced breast cancer in combination with paclitaxel did

not show improvement in PFS. Trial was stopped at the end of phase 2.
(Martín et al., 2017)

Cabozantinib

- **Alias:** XL-184
- **Brand Name:** Cometriq (for MTC); Cabometyx (for HCC and RCC)
- **Type Mechanism:** Potent inhibitor of RTKs, including AXL, FLT3, KIT, MET, RET, TIE-2, TRKB, and VEGFR1, VEGFR2, and VEGFR3. It induces apoptosis of cancer cells and suppresses tumor growth, metastasis, and angiogenesis.
- **Drug Class:** Multikinase inhibitor
- **Mechanism of Action:** Multikinase inhibitor
- **FDA Approval Date:** November 29, 2012
- **Indications:** Advanced HCC and RCC; metastatic MTC
- **Dose:** HCC dosing: 60 mg PO daily; RCC dosing: 40 mg PO daily with nivolumab or 60 mg PO daily (monotherapy); MTC dosing: 140 mg PO daily
- **Half-life:** Cometriq = ~55 hours; Cabometyx = ~99 hours
- **Metabolism:** Major CYP3A4 substrate
- **Side Effects:** Hemorrhage, perforation/fistula (U.S. box warning), HTN, stomatitis, palmar–plantar erythrodysesthesia, decreased appetite, weight loss, nausea/vomiting, diarrhea, tiredness and weakness, change in hair color, liver dysfunction (hyperbilirubinemia, transaminitis, increases alkaline phosphatase)
- **Clinical Pearls:** May affect the rate of wound healing; patients should notify doctor before surgery or dental work; moderate-to-high emetogenicity.

Camrelizumab

- **Alias:** SHR-1211
- **Type Mechanism:** An mAb directed against PD-1 (PCD-1) that binds to and blocks the binding of PD-1, expressed on activated T lymphocytes, B cells, and NK cells, to its ligands PD-L1, overexpressed on certain cancer cells, and PD-L2, which is primarily expressed on antigen-presenting cells (APCs). This prevents the activation of PD-1 and its downstream signaling pathways. Activation of CTLs and cell-mediated immune responses against tumor cells or pathogens.
- **Drug Class:** Checkpoint inhibitor
- **Mechanism of Action:** Monoclonal PD-1 inhibitor

- **Phase:** Phase 2/3
- **Indications:** Advanced SCC, NSCLC, HCC, advanced cervical cancer, and Hodgkin lymphoma
- **Dose:** 200 mg IV Q 2 weeks
- **Half-life:** 3 to 11 days
- **Side Effects:** Hyperbilirubinemia, stomatitis, anemia, diarrhea, increased ALT/AST, leukopenia, thrombocytopenia, rash, hyponatremia, hypochloremia

(Jackson et al., 2018)

Capivasertib

- **Alias:** AZD5363
- **Type Mechanism:** A novel pyrrolopyrimidine derivative and an inhibitor of the serine/threonine protein kinase AKT (protein kinase B) that binds to and inhibits all AKT isoforms. Inhibition of AKT prevents the phosphorylation of AKT substrates that mediate cellular processes, such as cell division, apoptosis, and glucose and fatty acid metabolism.
- **Drug Class:** Oral AKT inhibitor
- **Phase:** Phase 3 in combination with fulvestrant in metastatic ER+/HER2− breast cancer; advanced/metastatic TNBC; phase 3 meningioma
- **Indications:** TNBC; ER+/HER2− metastatic breast cancer

- **Dose:** RP2D: 480 mg PO BID for 4 days on, 3 days off for 21 days
- **Half-life:** 10 hours (range 7–15 hours)
- **Side Effects:** Maculopapular rash, hyperglycemia, diarrhea, nausea, neutropenia, fatigue

(Smyth et al., 2020)

Cediranib Maleate

- **Alias:** AZD 2171
- **Brand Name:** Recentin (tentative trade name)
- **Type Mechanism:** A potent VEGF RTK inhibitor of all three VEGF receptors (VEGFR1, VEGFR2, and VEGFR3). Inhibition of VEGF signaling leads to the inhibition of angiogenesis, lymphangiogenesis, neovascular survival, and vascular permeability. Cediranib also inhibits c-Kit tyrosine kinase.
- **Drug Class:** VEGFR inhibitor
- **Phase:** Phase 2/3; phase 3 monotherapy versus lomustine combination did not show PFS benefit.
- **Indications:** Advanced ovarian cancer with platinum resistance, fallopian tube cancer, and peritoneal cancer; mCRC
- **Dose:** 30 or 45 mg PO daily (20 mg when combined with cytotoxic chemotherapy)
- **Half-life:** 12 to 35 hours

- **Side Effects:** Fatigue, diarrhea, nausea, dysphonia, HTN (proteinuria), neutropenia

(Batchelor et al., 2013)

Ceritinib

- **Alias:** LDK378
- **Brand Name:** Zykadia
- **Type Mechanism:** An orally available inhibitor of the RTK activity of ALK that binds to and inhibits WT ALK, ALK fusion proteins, and ALK point mutation variants. Inhibition of ALK leads to both the disruption of ALK-mediated signaling and the inhibition of cell growth in ALK-overexpressing tumor cells.
- **Drug Class:** ALK inhibitor
- **FDA Approval Date:** April 29, 2014
- **Indications:** Metastatic NSCLC with ALK-positive mutation
- **Dose:** 450 mg PO daily with food
- **Half-life:** 41 hours
- **Metabolism:** Major CYP3A4 substrate and major CYP3A4 inhibitor
- **Side Effects:** QT prolongation, nausea/vomiting, abdominal pain, diarrhea, neuropathy, fatigue, skin rash, hyperglycemia, increased lipase, transaminitis, hyperbilirubinemia, visual impairment

Cetuximab

- **Alias:** C225; IMC-C225
- **Brand Name:** Erbitux
- **Type Mechanism:** A recombinant human/mouse chimeric mAb that binds specifically to EGFR (HER1, c-ErbB-1) and competitively inhibits the binding of EGF and other ligands
- **Drug Class:** EGFR inhibitor
- **FDA Approval Date:** February 12, 2004
- **Indications:** KRAS WT CRC; SCCHN; off label for RAS WT, BRAF V600E–mutated CRC, SCC of the penis, and SCC of the skin
- **Dose:** Weekly dose: 400 mg/m^2 as 120-minute IV infusion as an initial dose, followed by 250 mg/m^2 infused over 30 minutes weekly. Biweekly dose: 500 mg/m^2 IV over 120 minutes once Q 2 weeks
- **Half-life:** ~112 hours
- **Side Effects:** Infusion reactions (U.S. box warning), nausea/vomiting, diarrhea, skin problems (acneiform rash, pruritus), hypomagnesemia, stomatitis, lung disease (dyspnea, cough), fatigue, neutropenia, transaminitis, palmar–plantar erythrodysesthesia, xeroderma
- **Clinical Pearls:** Severity of acneiform rash can be minimized with the use of topical steroid cream, topical antibiotic gel, and doxycycline.

Cixutumumab

- **Alias:** IMC-A12; CIX
- **Type Mechanism:** A fully human IgG1/λ mAb directed at the IGF-IR
  - Has a dual action of inhibiting the binding of IGF-1 and IGF-2 ligands to the IGF-1R and inducing the rapid internalization of the receptor
- **Drug Class:** IGF-1R inhibitor
- **Phase:** Phase 2
- **Indications:** Breast cancer, rhabdomyosarcoma, Ewing sarcoma, NSCLC, pancreatic carcinoma, adrenocortical carcinoma, metastatic prostate cancer, and HCC
- **Dose:** 6 to 10 mg/kg IV Q 1 to 2 weeks
- **Half-life:** 148 to 209 hours
- **Side Effects:** Hyperglycemia, rash, pruritis, fatigue, nephrotoxicity, diarrhea, mucositis, lymphopenia, hypophosphatemia, anemia, neutropenia, hyperlipidemia

(Higano et al., 2007)

Cobimetinib Fumarate

- **Alias:** GDC-0973; XL518
- **Brand Name:** Cotellic
- **Type Mechanism:** An orally bioavailable small-molecule inhibitor of MAP2K1 or MEK1 that specifically binds to and inhibits the catalytic activity of MEK1, resulting in the inhibition of ERK2 phosphorylation and activation and reduced tumor cell proliferation
- **Drug Class:** MEK inhibitor
- **FDA Approval Date:** March 28, 2016
- **Indications:** Unresectable or metastatic melanoma with BRAF V600E or V600K mutation in combination with vemurafenib
- **Dose:** 60 mg daily for 21 days of the 28-day cycle
- **Half-life:** Average 44 hours (range 23–70 hours)
- **Metabolism:** Major CYP3A4 substrate
- **Side Effects:** Decreased LVEF; HTN; photosensitivity; ocular toxicities such as serous retinopathy, chorioretinopathy, and retinal detachment; acneiform eruption; hypophosphatemia; increased GGT; nausea/vomiting; diarrhea; anemia; transaminitis; visual impairment; increased SCr

Copanlisib

- **Alias:** BAY 80-6946
- **Brand Name:** Aliqopa
- **Type Mechanism:** Inhibits PI3K, primarily the P13K-α and P13K-δ isoforms that are expressed in malignant B cells. It induces tumor cell death through apoptosis and inhibition of proliferation of primary

malignant B-cell lines. It also inhibits several signaling pathways, including BCR signaling, CXCR12-mediated chemotaxis of malignant B cells, and NFκB signaling in lymphoma cell lines.

- **FDA Approval Date:** September 14, 2017
- **Indications:** Relapsed FL
- **Dose:** 60 mg IV on days 1, 8, and 15 of a 28-day cycle
- **Half-life:** 39.1 hours (range 14.6–82.4 hours)
- **Metabolism:** Major CYP3A4 substrate; if potent CYP3A4 inhibitors cannot be avoided, may decrease dose of copanlisib to 45 mg
- **Side Effects:** Hyperglycemia, nausea/diarrhea, mucositis, fatigue, HTN, skin rash, hypertriglyceridemia, hypophosphatemia

Crizotinib

- **Brand Name:** Xalkori
- **Type Mechanism:** A tyrosine kinase receptor inhibitor that inhibits ALK, HGFR (c-MET), ROS1 (c-ros), and recepteur d'origine nantais (RON). It induces apoptosis and inhibits proliferation and ALK-mediated signaling in ALCL-derived cell lines.
- **FDA Approval Date:** August 26, 2011
- **Indications:** Locally advanced or metastatic ALK-positive NSCLC
- **Dose:** 250 mg PO BID

- **Half-life:** 42 hours
- **Metabolism:** Major CYP3A4 substrate and P-glycoprotein; moderate CYP3A4 inhibitor
- **Side Effects:** Edema, vision problems (diplopia, blurred vision), nausea/vomiting, diarrhea, dysphagia, GERD, reflux esophagitis, skin rash, swelling of hands and feet, fatigue, dizziness, transaminitis
- **Clinical Pearls:** Advise patients to exercise, caution when driving or operating machinery because of the risk of developing visual changes such as floaters, blurred vision, light sensitivity, or flashes of light.

Dabrafenib

- **Alias:** GSK2118436
- **Brand Name:** Tafinlar
- **Type Mechanism:** Selectively binds to and inhibits the activity of B-raf, which may inhibit the proliferation of tumor cells that contain a mutated *BRAF* gene
- **FDA Approval Date:** March 29, 2013
- **Indications:** Melanoma with BRAF V600E or V600K; metastatic NSCLC with BRAF V600E; metastatic, anaplastic thyroid cancer with BRAF V600E in combination with trametinib

- **Dose:** 150 mg PO BID on fasting stomach at least 1 hour before or 2 hours after meals
- **Half-life:** Parent drug 8 hours; hydroxy-dabrafenib (active metabolite) 10 hours; desmethyl-dabrafenib (active metabolite) 21 to 22 hours
- **Metabolism:** Major CYP2C8 and CYP3A4 substrates; moderate CYP3A4 inducer
- **Side Effects:** Keratoacanthoma and SCC, fatigue, arthralgias, pyrexia, papilloma, hyperglycemia, hyperkeratosis, palmar–plantar erythrodysesthesia, skin rash, hypophosphatemia
- **Clinical Pearls:** Corticosteroids may be used as an effective fever prophylaxis when fever occurs.

Dacomitinib

- **Alias:** PF-00299804
- **Brand Name:** Vizimpro
- **Type Mechanism:** Second-generation small-molecule inhibitor of the pan-EGFR family of tyrosine kinases (ErbB family) that binds to and inhibits human EGFR subtypes, resulting in inhibition of proliferation and induction of apoptosis in EGFR-expressing tumor cells
- **FDA Approval Date:** September 27, 2018
- **Indications:** First-line EGFR exon 19 del, or exon 21 L858 substitution mutation–positive NSCLC
- **Dose:** 45 mg PO once daily with or without food
- **Half-life:** 70 hours
- **Metabolism:** Major CYP2D6 inhibitor; weak CYP2D6 substrate
- **Side Effects:** Diarrhea, dermatitis acneiform (dry skin), stomatitis, paronychia, liver dysfunction (increased bilirubin, ALT/AST), palmar–plantar erythrodysesthesia, pruritus, skin rash, anemia, limb pain

Dactolisib

- **Alias:** BEZ235; NVP-BEZ235
- **Type Mechanism:** An imidazoquinoline that acts as a dual ATP-competitive PI3K and mTOR inhibitor for p110α/γ/δ/β and mTOR(p70S6K)
- **Drug Class:** PI3K/mTOR inhibitor
- **Phase:** Phase 1b
- **Indications:** pNETs
- **Dose:** 400 to 800 mg PO daily (in combination with everolimus). Taken with food/breakfast. No Seville orange juice or grapefruit juice
- **Half-life:** 15 to 43 hours
- **Metabolism:** Time-dependent CYP3A4 inhibitor

- **Side Effects:** Nausea/vomiting, fatigue, asthenia, anemia, anorexia, diarrhea, mucositis, myelosuppression, transaminitis

(Wise-Draper et al., 2017)

Danvatirsen

- **Alias:** AZD9150; IONIS-STAT3-2.5; ISIS 481464
- **Type Mechanism:** An antisense oligonucleotide targeting STAT3, leading to apoptosis and reduced tumor cell growth
- **Mechanism of Action:** Generation 2.5 antisense therapy targeting STAT3
- **Phase:** Phase 2 in NSCLC, bladder cancer, head and neck (H&N) cancer, diffuse large B-cell lymphoma (DLBCL), and AML
- **Indications:** SCCHN, NSCLC, bladder cancer, and relapsed/refractory DLBCL
- **Dose:** RP2D: 200 mg (flat dose) IV Q week
- **Half-life:** 20 days
- **Side Effects:** Thrombocytopenia, transaminitis

(Xu et al., 2019)

Darolutamide

- **Alias:** ODM-201; BAY-1841788
- **Brand Name:** Nubeqa
- **Type Mechanism:** An AR antagonist that can also inhibit the transcriptional activity of several AR mutant variants (F877L, F877L/T878A, and H875Y/T878A), which are enzalutamide resistant. It inhibits androgen-induced receptor activation, thus facilitating the formation of inactive complexes that cannot translocate to the nucleus. This prevents binding to and transcription of AR-responsive genes that regulate prostate cancer cell proliferation.
- **Drug Class:** AR antagonist
- **FDA Approval Date:** July 30, 2019
- **Indications:** Non-MCRPC
- **Dose:** 600 mg PO BID (usually in combination with GnRH analog)
- **Half-life:** ~20 hours
- **Metabolism:** Weak CYP3A4 substrate; UGT1A1 and UGT1A9 substrate; BCRP/ABCG2 inhibitor, OATP1B1/1B3 inhibitor
- **Side Effects:** Fatigue, neutropenia, AST elevation, hyperbilirubinemia, asthenia, skin rash

Debio-1347

- **Type Mechanism:** An orally bioavailable inhibitor of the FGFR1/2/3 that binds to and inhibits FGFR1, FGFR2, and FGFR3, which result in the inhibition of FGFR-mediated signal transduction pathways. This leads to the inhibition of both tumor cell proliferation and angiogenesis and causes cell death in FGFR-overexpressing tumor cells.

- **Drug Class:** FGFR inhibitor
- **Phase:** Phase 1/2
- **Indications:** All solid tumors harboring *FGFR1-3* gene fusion
- **Dose:** P2RD: 80 mg PO daily
- **Half-life:** 11.5 hours
- **Side Effects:** Fatigue, hyperphosphatemia, anemia, alopecia, nausea/vomiting, constipation, palmar–plantar erythrodysesthesia syndrome, minor blurred vision (dry eyes), xerostomia, hyperbilirubinemia, stomatitis

(Cleary et al., 2020)

Dostarlimab

- **Alias:** TSR-042; ANB011
- **Brand Name:** Jemperli
- **Type Mechanism:** An anti–PD-1 humanized IgG4 mAb that inhibits PD-1 activity by binding to the PD-1 receptor on T cells to block PD-1 ligands (PD-L1 and PD-L2) from binding
- **Drug Class:** Anti–PD-1 mAb
- **FDA Approval Date:** April 22, 2021
- **Indications:** Recurrent or advanced endometrial cancer with the presence of deficient mismatch repair (dMMR) in tumor specimen
- **Dose:** 500 mg IV Q 3 weeks for 4 doses, then 1,000 mg IV Q 6 weeks for 5 doses or more. Dose #5 should begin 3 weeks after dose #4.
- **Half-life:** 25.4 days
- **Side Effects:** Pruritus, hypercalcemia, diarrhea, nausea/vomiting, anemia, leukopenia, transaminitis, fatigue, myalgias, asthenia, increased SCr

---

Dovitinib

- **Alias:** TKI258, CHIR-258
- **Type Mechanism:** A benzimidazole–quinolinone compound strongly binds to fibroblast growth factor receptor 3 (FGFR3) and inhibits its phosphorylation, which may result in the inhibition of tumor cell proliferation and the induction of tumor cell death. It also inhibits other members of the RTK superfamily, including the VEGFR; FGFR1; PDGFR type 3; FMS-like tyrosine kinase 3; stem cell factor receptor (c-KIT); and colony-stimulating factor receptor 1
- **Drug Class:** Multitargeted RTK inhibitor

- **Phase:** Phase 2
- **Indications (1):** Metastatic renal cell carcinoma, HR+, HER2− breast cancer, metastatic adenoid cystic carcinoma, GIST, and advanced/metastatic thyroid cancer
- **Dose:** 500 mg orally once daily (5 days on/2 days off)
- **Half-life:** 13 hours
- **Metabolism:** CYP1A2 inducer
- **Side Effects:** Fatigue, diarrhea, nausea/vomiting, decreased appetite, asthenia, headache, acneiform rash, hypertriglyceridemia, neutropenia, thrombocytopenia

---

Durvalumab

- **Alias:** MEDI4736
- **Brand Name:** Imfinzi
- **Type Mechanism:** A human IgG1κ mAb that blocks PD-L1 binding to PD-1 and CD80 (B7.1); PD-L1 blockade leads to increased T-cell activation, allowing T cells to kill tumor cells. PD-L1 is an immune checkpoint protein expressed on tumor cells and tumor-infiltrating cells and downregulates antitumor T-cell function by binding to PD-1 and B7.1; blocking PD-1 and B7.1 interactions restores antitumor T-cell function.

- **Drug Class:** Anti–PD-L1 mAb
- **FDA Approval Date:** May 1, 2017
- **Indications:** Unresectable NSCLC and extensive stage SCLC; locally advanced or metastatic urothelial carcinoma
- **Dose:** 10 mg/kg IV Q 2 weeks; may use flat dosing of 1,500 mg IV Q 3 to 4 weeks for patients ≥30 kg
- **Half-life:** ~18 days
- **Side Effects:** Fatigue, skin rash, muscle pain, peripheral edema, abdominal pain, lymphocytopenia, constipation, immune-mediated pneumonitis

---

Elacestrant

- **Alias:** RAD1901
- **Manufacturer:** Radius
- **Type Mechanism:** nonsteroidal, selective estrogen receptor degrader
- **Drug Class:** Anti-estrogen
- **Trials:** Ongoing Phase 2 and 3 trials
- **Indications:** Metastatic breast cancer with *ESR1* mutations (FDA fast track designation for HR-positive MBC who harbor ESR1 mutations)
- **Dose:** 400 mg oral daily
- **Half-life:** 27–47 hours

- **Metabolism:** CYP3A4 interaction
- **Side Effects:** nausea/vomiting, hypophosphatemia, hypertriglyceridemia, decreased appetite, diarrhea, fatigue, back pain

Enasidenib Mesylate

- **Alias:** AG-221; CC-90007
- **Brand Name:** Idhifa
- **Type Mechanism:** A small-molecule inhibitor of the enzyme isocitrate dehydrogenase 2 (IDH2) that targets the mutant IDH2 variants R140Q, R172S, and R172K. Mutant IDH2 inhibition results in decreased 2HG levels, reduced abnormal histone hypermethylation, and restored myeloid differentiation. It also reduces blast counts and increases percentages of mature myeloid cells.
- **Drug Class:** IDH2 inhibitor
- **FDA Approval Date:** August 1, 2017
- **Indications:** Relapsed/refractory ALL with IDH2 mutation
- **Dose:** 100 mg PO daily until disease progression (PD)
- **Half-life:** 7.9 days
- **Metabolism:** Minor CYP1A2, CYP2B6, CYP2C19, CYP2C8, CYP2D6, CYP3A4, UGT1A1, UGT1A3, UGT1A4 substrates; BCRP/ABCG2 inhibitor; OATP1B1/1B3 inhibitor
- **Side Effects:** Hypocalcemia, hypokalemia, nausea, diarrhea, decreased appetite, dysgeusia, hyperbilirubinemia, CRS, TLS

Encorafenib

- **Alias:** LGX818
- **Brand Name:** Braftovi
- **Type Mechanism:** An ATP-competitive inhibitor of protein kinase B-raf (BRAF) that suppresses the MAPK pathway and targets BRAF V600E, V600 D, and V600 K. It has a longer dissociation half-life than other BRAF inhibitors, allowing for sustained inhibition. BRAF V600 mutations result in constitutive activation of the BRAF pathway (which may stimulate tumor growth); BRAF inhibition inhibits tumor cell growth.
- **Drug Class:** BRAF inhibitor
- **FDA Approval Date:** April 8, 2020
- **Indications:** Metastatic, BRAF V600E–mutant CRC and unresectable/metastatic BRAF V600E– or V600K-mutated melanoma
- **Dose:** CRC: 300 mg PO daily with cetuximab; melanoma: 450 mg PO daily with binimetinib
- **Half-life:** 3.5 hours

- **Metabolism:** Major CYP3A4 substrate
- **Side Effects:** Anemia, hyperglycemia, fever, increased lipase, HTN, fatigue, nausea, arthralgia, palmar–plantar erythrodysesthesia, acneiform eruption, alopecia, hyperkeratosis, xeroderma, arthralgia, increased SCr

Entrectinib

- **Alias:** RXDX-101
- **Brand Name:** Rozlytrek
- **Type Mechanism:** Inhibits TRK receptors such as TRKA, TRKB, and TRKC. TRKA, TRKB, and TRKC are encoded by NTRK genes *NTRK1*, *NTRK2*, and *NTRK3*, respectively. It also inhibits proto-oncogenic tyrosine protein kinase ROS1 and ALK. M5 (the major active entrectinib metabolite) demonstrated similar activity (in vitro) against TRK, ROS1, and ALK. Fusion proteins that include TRK, ROS1, or ALK domains act as oncogenic drivers to promote hyperactivation of downstream signaling pathways, resulting in unchecked cell proliferation.
- **Drug Class:** TRK inhibitor
- **FDA Approval Date:** August 15, 2019
- **Indications:** Metastatic NSCLC with ROS1 positive; all metastatic, unresectable solid tumors with *NTRK* gene fusion
- **Dose:** 600 mg PO daily
- **Half-life:** Entrectinib = 20 hours
  - M5 active metabolite = 40 hours
- **Metabolism:** Major CYP3A4 substrate
- **Side Effects:** Edema, hypotension, fatigue, cognitive dysfunction, sleep disorder, myasthenia, hyperuricemia, dysgeusia, constipation, diarrhea, increased lipase, anemia, lymphocytopenia, neutropenia myalgia, arthralgia, visual disturbance, elevated SCr, cough, fever
- **Clinical Pearls:** Avoid grapefruit or grapefruit juice as it may increase the levels of entrectinib.

Enzalutamide

- **Alias:** MDV-3100
- **Brand Name:** Xtandi
- **Type Mechanism:** A pure AR signaling inhibitor with no known agonistic properties. It inhibits AR nuclear translocation, DNA binding, and coactivator mobilization, leading to cellular apoptosis and decreased prostate tumor volume.
- **Drug Class:** AR signaling inhibitor
- **FDA Approval Date:** August 31, 2012
- **Indications:** MCRPC
- **Dose:** 160 mg PO daily

- **Half-life:** Parent drug = 5.8 days
  - *N*-Desmethyl enzalutamide = 7.8 to 8.6 days
- **Metabolism:** Major CYP2C8 and CYP3A4 substrates; moderate CYP2C19 and CYP2C9 inducers; major CYP3A4 inducer
- **Side Effects:** Peripheral edema, HTN, fatigue, hot flashes, back pain/arthralgia, URI, neutropenia, hyperglycemia, nausea, neutropenia, dyspnea

Erdafitinib

- **Alias:** JNJ-42756493
- **Brand Name:** Balversa
- **Type Mechanism:** A pan-FGFR kinase inhibitor that binds to and inhibits FGFR1, FGFR2, FGFR3, and FGFR4 enzyme activity. Erdafitinib also binds to RET, CSF1R, PDGFRα, PDGFRβ, FLT4, KIT, and VEGFR2. FGFR inhibition results in decreased FGFR-related signaling and decreased cell viability in cell lines expressing FGFR genetic alterations, including point mutations, amplifications, and fusions.
- **Drug Class:** FGFR inhibitor
- **FDA Approval Date:** April 14, 2019
- **Indications:** Advanced/metastatic urothelial carcinoma with susceptible FGFR genetic alteration

- **Dose:** 8 mg PO daily for 14 days; if serum phosphate ≤5.5 mg/dL, and no ocular toxicity ≥ grade 2 common terminology criteria for adverse events (CTCAEs), then increase dose 9 mg PO daily.
- **Half-life:** 59 hours
- **Metabolism:** Major CYP2C9 and CYP3A4 substrates
- **Side Effects:** Fatigue, onycholysis, xeroderma, alopecia, palmar–plantar erythrodysesthesia, paronychia, nail discoloration, hyperphosphatemia, hyponatremia, stomatitis, diarrhea, xerostomia, dysgeusia, anemia, thrombocytopenia, leukopenia, transaminitis, dry eyes syndrome, central serous retinopathy, blurred vision, elevated SCr, myalgia

Erlotinib

- **Alias:** OSI-774; CP 358774
- **Brand Name:** Tarceva
- **Type Mechanism:** Reversibly binds to the intracellular catalytic domain of EGFR and inhibits overall HER1/EGFR tyrosine kinase. Active competitive inhibition of ATP inhibits downstream signal transduction of ligand-dependent HER1/EGFR activation.
- **Drug Class:** EGFR inhibitor

- **FDA Approval Date:** November 18, 2004
- **Indications:** Metastatic NSCLC with EGFR exon 19 deletions or exon 21 substitution mutations; locally advanced, unresectable, or metastatic pancreatic cancer (in combination with gemcitabine); off-label use for advanced papillary RCC
- **Dose:** 150 mg once daily (NSCLC) and 100 mg once daily (pancreatic cancer) on empty stomach 1 hour before or 2 hours after meals
- **Half-life:** 36 hours
- **Metabolism:** Major CYP3A4 and CYP1A2 substrates
- **Side Effects:** Rash (acne vulgaris, pruritus), diarrhea, paronychia (hair and nail changes), fatigue, weakness, back pain, cough, dyspnea, conjunctivitis, chest pain, xeroderma, anorexia, nausea, mucositis, dry eyes syndrome, increased ALT and GGT
- **Clinical Pearls:** Severity of acne-form rash can be minimized with the use of topical steroid cream, topical antibiotic gel, and doxycycline; encourage smoking cessation before start because smoking can make the drug less effective.

Everolimus

- **Alias:** RAD001
- **Brand Name:** Afinitor

- **Type Mechanism:** An mTOR inhibitor that has antiproliferative and antiangiogenic properties. Reduces protein synthesis and cell proliferation by binding to the FKBP-12, an intracellular protein, to form a complex that inhibits activation of mTOR serine-threonine kinase activity. Also reduces angiogenesis by inhibiting VEGF and hypoxia-inducible factor (HIF-1) expression.
- **Drug Class:** mTOR inhibitor
- **FDA Approval Date:** March 30, 2009
- **Indications:** Advanced RCC, neuroendocrine carcinomas (GI, lung, or pancreatic origin), and advanced, HR+, HER2− breast cancer in combination with exemestane; off-label use in advanced carcinoid tumors, relapsed/refractory Hodgkin lymphoma, advanced/refractory thymoma and thymic carcinoma
- **Dose:** 10 mg once daily with or without food. Dosing with 5 mg if combined with lenvatinib for RCC
- **Half-life:** 30 hours
- **Metabolism:** Major CYP3A4 substrate and P-glycoprotein substrate
- **Side Effects:** Mouth ulcers, rash (acneiform), delayed wound healing, nausea/vomiting, fatigue, anorexia (decreased appetite), cough, shortness of breath, thrombocytopenia,

diarrhea or constipation,
hypercholesterolemia, HTN,
hyperglycemia, anemia,
leukopenia
- **Clinical Pearls:** Monitor fasting triglycerides and cholesterol. Levels may increase while on treatment despite the patient's dietary habits. Initiate oral care early on (soft toothbrush, salt, and soda swish).

Farletuzumab

- **Alias:** MORAb-003
- **Type Mechanism:** An mAb to folate receptor α that leads to cell-mediated cytotoxicity, complement-dependent killing, and inhibition of growth under limited folate conditions
- **Drug Class:** Folate receptor α inhibitor
- **Phase:** Phase 2/3
- **Indications:** Platinum-sensitive ovarian cancer
- **Dose:** 1.25 or 2.5 mg/kg IV Q week in combination with chemotherapy
- **Half-life:** 56 to 260 hours (increased with dose and multiple infusions)
- **Side Effects:** Fatigue, nausea, drug hypersensitivity, headache, cough, exertional dyspnea

(Konner et al., 2010)

Figitumumab

- **Alias:** CP-751871
- **Type Mechanism:** A human mAb directed against the IGF-1R. Selectively binds to IGF-1R to prevent IGF1 from binding to the receptor and subsequent receptor autophosphorylation
- **Mechanism of Action:** Phase 3 trial for advanced NSCLC failed to show any benefits.
- **Phase:** Currently, no active clinical trials in the United States. Failed to meet the end point of phase 3 trial
- **Dose:** 20 mg/kg IV (day 1 of a 21-day cycle)
- **Half-life:** 3 weeks
- **Side Effects:** Hyperglycemia, nausea/vomiting, muscle cramps, fatigue, anorexia, increased GGT

(Langer et al., 2014)

Foretinib

- **Alias:** GSK1363089; XL880
- **Type Mechanism:** Binds to and selectively inhibits MET and VEGFR2
- **Mechanism of Action:** Phase 2 clinical trials discontinued on October 2015
- **Phase:** Currently under investigation in phase 2 clinical trial for SCCHN, metastatic gastric cancer, papillary RCC, and nonsarcomatous GEJ adenocarcinoma

- **Indications:** SCCHN, metastatic gastric cancer, papillary RCC, and nonsarcomatous GEJ adenocarcinoma
- **Dose:** 240 mg PO daily for 5 days Q 14 days
- **Half-life:** 40 hours
- **Side Effects:** Fatigue, nausea/vomiting, diarrhea, HTN, proteinuria, increased lipase, increased AST

(Choueiri et al., 2013)

Fulvestrant

- **Alias:** ICI-182,780; ZD9238
- **Brand Name:** Faslodex
- **Type Mechanism:** An estrogen receptor antagonist; competitively binds to estrogen receptors on tumors and other tissue targets, producing a nuclear complex that causes a dose-related downregulation of estrogen receptors and inhibits tumor growth
- **Drug Class:** Estrogen receptor antagonist
- **FDA Approval Date:** April 25, 2002
- **Indications:** HR-positive and/or HER2-negative breast cancer as monotherapy or combination therapy (e.g., CDK inhibitors)
- **Dose:** 500 mg intramuscularly (IM) on days 1, 15, and 29 with 500 mg IM monthly maintenance
- **Half-life:** ~40 days

- **Metabolism:** Minor CYP3A4
- **Side Effects:** Decreased serum glucose, hot flash, GGT elevation, transaminitis with ALT/AST elevations, diarrhea, abdominal pain, stomatitis, nausea, fatigue, headache, arthralgia
- **Clinical Pearls:** LHRH agonist should be administered to pre-/perimenopausal women in combination with CDK inhibitors.

Futibatinib

- **Alias:** TAS-120
- **Type Mechanism:** An orally bioavailable inhibitor of the FGFR that selectively and irreversibly binds to and inhibits FGFR, which may result in the inhibition of both the FGFR-mediated signal transduction pathway and tumor cell proliferation and increased cell death in FGFR-overexpressing tumor cells. FGFR is an RTK essential to tumor cell proliferation, differentiation, and survival, and its expression is upregulated in many tumor cell types.
- **Drug Class:** FGFR inhibitor
- **Phase:** Phase 3
- **Indications:** Advanced cholangiocarcinoma harboring *FGFR2* gene rearrangements
- **Dose:** 20 mg PO daily

- **Half-life:** ~3 hours
- **Metabolism:** Major CYP3A4 substrate; P-glycoprotein/BCRP substrate
- **Side Effects:** Stomatitis, oral dysesthesia, transaminitis, diarrhea, hyperphosphatemia, constipation, hyperbilirubinemia, hyponatremia, increased lipase, increased CPK, dry mouth, decreased appetite

(Chatila et al., 2020)

Galunisertib

- **Alias:** LY2157299
- **Type Mechanism:** An orally available, small-molecule antagonist of the tyrosine kinase TGF-β receptor type 1 (TGFβR1) that specifically targets and binds to the kinase domain of TGFβR1, thereby preventing the activation of TGF-β–mediated signaling pathways. This may inhibit the proliferation of TGF-β–overexpressing tumor cells.
- **Phase:** Phase 1b/2
- **Indications:** Advanced HCC; unresectable, advanced pancreatic cancer
- **Dose:** 150 mg PO BID for 14 days on, 14 days off for a 28-day cycle
- **Half-life:** 8 hours

- **Side Effects:** Fatigue, thrombosis, dyspnea, thrombocytopenia, lymphopenia, anemia, neutropenia, increased bilirubin, hypoalbuminemia, peripheral edema

(Kelley et al., 2019)

Ganitumab

- **Alias:** AMG 479
- **Type Mechanism:** A recombinant fully human mAb that binds to membrane-bound IGF-1R, subsequently inhibiting cancer cell proliferation through disruption of the PI3K/AKT and MAPK pathways
- **Drug Class:** EGFR inhibitor
- **Phase:** Phase 2/3; granted orphan drug status for Ewing sarcoma in April 2017
- **Indications:** Metastatic Ewing sarcoma, mutant KRAS mCRC in combination with FOLFIRI, metastatic pancreatic cancer
- **Dose:** 12 mg/kg IV Q 2 weeks in combination with cytotoxic chemotherapy or targeted therapy
- **Half-life:** 7 days
- **Side Effects:** Hyperglycemia, fatigue, nausea/vomiting, anorexia, neutropenia, thrombocytopenia, increased AST

(Tap et al., 2012)

Gefitinib

- **Alias:** ZD1839
- **Brand Name:** Iressa
- **Type Mechanism:** A TKI that reversibly inhibits kinase activity of WT and select activation mutations of EGFR. It prevents autophosphorylation of tyrosine residues associated with the EGFR, which blocks downstream signaling and EGFR-dependent proliferation. Gefitinib has a higher binding affinity for EGFR exon 19 deletion and exon 21 (L858R) substitution mutation than for WT EGFR.
- **Drug Class:** EGFR inhibitor
- **FDA Approval Date:** July 14, 2015
- **Indications:** First-line treatment for metastatic NSCLC with EGFR exon 19 deletions or exon 21 (L858R) substitution mutations
- **Dose:** 250 mg PO once daily with or without food
- **Half-life:** 48 hours
- **Metabolism:** Major CYP3A4 substrate; BCRP/ABCG2 substrate
- **Side Effects:** Skin rash (dry skin), nausea/vomiting, diarrhea, anorexia, pruritus, fatigue, acne vulgaris, stomatitis, ALT/AST elevation

Geldanamycin

- **Alias:** Tanespimycin (17AAG)
- **Type Mechanism:** Inhibits the ATPase activity of chaperone heat shock protein 90 (Hsp90), which maintains conformation, stability, and function of oncogenic protein kinases involved in signal transduction cascades, leading to proliferation and progression of cell cycle and apoptosis
- **Drug Class:** Benzoquinone ansamycin HSP90 inhibitors
- **Phase:** Phase 2
- **Indications:** Phase 2 in metastatic pancreatic cancer, metastatic melanoma, EGFR-mutated NSCLC, metastatic breast cancer
- **Dose:** RP2D: 220 mg/m^2 IV on days 1, 4, 8, and 11 of a 21-day cycle
- **Half-life:** 3.8 to 8.6 hours
- **Side Effects:** Diarrhea, transaminitis, hyperbilirubinemia, anorexia, fatigue, nausea, pleural effusion

(Gartner et al., 2012)

Iniparib

- **Alias:** BSI-201
- **Type Mechanism:** A small-molecule iodobenzamide that has shown to have

anticancer activity through a prodrug mechanism in which an active nitro radical ion is released through one- and two-electron cytosolic activation, rather than direct PARP inhibition

- **Phase:** Phase 2
- **Indications:** Malignant gliomas in combination with RT and temozolomide
- **Dose:** 8.6 mg/kg IV TIW for 6 cycles
- **Half-life:** Iniparib = 11 minutes; active metabolite IABM = 0.8 hours; and active metabolite IABA = 2.1 hours
- **Metabolism:** Nitro reduction pathway
- **Side Effects:** Fatigue, rash, thrombocytopenia, neutropenia, elevated ALT/AST, hyperbilirubinemia, abdominal pain, diarrhea, nausea, anorexia
- **Clinical Pearls:** Trials in phase 3 TNBC and squamous cell lung cancer and phase 2 in platinum-resistant ovarian cancer failed to show survival benefit. On June 2013, manufacture dropped the development of drug.

(Blakeley et al., 2019)

Ipatasertib

- **Alias:** GDC-0068; RG-7440
- **Type Mechanism:** An inhibitor of the serine/threonine protein kinase Akt (protein kinase B) that binds to and inhibits the activity of Akt in a non–ATP-competitive manner, which may result in the inhibition of the PI3K/Akt signaling pathway and tumor cell proliferation and the induction of tumor cell apoptosis
- **Drug Class:** AKT inhibitor
- **Phase:** Phase 2
- **Indications:** Metastatic prostate cancer with and without PTEN loss in combination with abiraterone
- **Dose:** 400 mg PO daily for 21 days on, 7 days off
- **Half-life:** 31.9 to 53 hours
- **Side Effects:** Diarrhea, nausea, vomiting, asthenia, rash, decreased appetite, hyperglycemia
- **Clinical Pearls:** Ipatunity-130 study failed both cohorts of TNBC and HR+ HER2− breast cancer.

(de Bono et al., 2019)

Ipilimumab

- **Alias:** MDX-010; MDX-CTLA-4
- **Brand Name:** Yervoy
- **Type Mechanism:** A recombinant human IgG1 mAb that binds to the CTLA4. CTLA4 is a downregulator of T-cell activation pathways. Blocking CTLA4 allows for enhanced T-cell activation and proliferation.

- **Drug Class:** Anti-CTLA4 mAb
- **FDA Approval Date:** March 25, 2011
- **Indications:** Microsatellite instability high (MSI-H) or dMMR mCRC; HCC (in combination with nivolumab); unresectable, malignant pleural mesothelioma; unresectable or metastatic melanoma (in combination with nivolumab); metastatic/recurrent NSCLC with no EGFR or ALK; advanced RCC (in combination with nivolumab)
- **Dose:** Range of dose from 1 mg/kg IV Q 3 weeks, 3 mg/kg IV Q 3 weeks, or 10 mg/kg IV Q 3 weeks, up to 4 doses; NSCLC dose = 1 mg/kg IV Q 6 weeks until PD
- **Half-life:** 15.4 days
- **Side Effects:** Immune-mediated adverse effects (TEN, endocrine disorder, enterocolitis, hepatitis, neuropathy) (black box warning), fatigue, headache, rash/pruritus, nausea/vomiting, diarrhea, abdominal pain, elevated amylase/lipase, elevated ALT/AST, hyperbilirubinemia

---

Ivosidenib

- **Alias:** AG-120
- **Brand Name:** Tibsovo
- **Type Mechanism:** An inhibitor of isocitrate dehydrogenase type 1 (IDH1) that inhibits a mutated form of IDH1 in the cytoplasm, which inhibits the formation of the oncometabolite, 2HG. This may lead to both an induction of cellular differentiation and an inhibition of cellular proliferation in IDH1-expressing tumor cells. IDH1, an enzyme in the citric acid cycle, is mutated in a variety of cancers; it initiates and drives cancer growth by both blocking cell differentiation and catalyzing the formation of 2HG.
- **Drug Class:** IDH1 inhibitor
- **FDA Approval Date:** July 20, 2018
- **Indications:** Relapsed/refractory or newly diagnosed AML in adults older than ≥75 years with IDH1 mutation
- **Dose:** 500 mg PO daily. Do not take with high-fat meals due to 98% increase in C_{max}.
- **Half-life:** 93 hours
- **Metabolism:** Major CYP3A4 substrate
- **Side Effects:** Fatigue, diarrhea, nausea, decreased appetite, peripheral edema, prolonged QTc, dyspnea, anemia, HTN, transaminitis, leukocytosis due to differentiation syndrome, abdominal pain, skin rash, pruritus
- **Clinical Pearls:** ClarIDHy phase 3 trial demonstrated compelling results for treatment with previously treated, IDH1-mutant cholangiocarcinoma.

Lapatinib Ditosylate

- **Alias:** GSK572016; GW2016; GW-572016
- **Brand Name:** Tykerb
- **Type Mechanism:** Reversibly blocks phosphorylation of the EGFR, HER2, and the ERK1, ERK2, and AKT kinases. Inhibits cyclin D protein levels in human tumor cell lines and xenografts
- **FDA Approval Date:** March 13, 2007
- **Indications:** Metastatic or advanced breast cancer with HER2 overexpression
- **Dose:** 1,250 mg once daily in combination with capecitabine 2,000 mg/m^2 daily, 1,500 mg once daily in combination with letrozole 2.5 mg once daily. Take 1 hour before or 1 hour after meals and avoid grapefruit juice.
- **Half-life:** 24 hours
- **Metabolism:** Major CYP3A4 and P-glycoprotein substrates
- **Side Effects:** Myelosuppression, hand-foot syndrome, liver dysfunction (increased bilirubin, transaminitis), fatigue, nausea/vomiting, diarrhea, rash, decreased LVEF
- **Clinical Pearls:** LVEF should be evaluated in patients before starting therapy, because a decreased EF can occur within the first 9 weeks of treatment. Oral steroids can decrease the levels of the drug and make it less effective. This drug can change the rhythm of the heart. Exercise caution with patients who are already on medications to control irregular heart rhythm.

Larotrectinib

- **Alias:** LOXO-101; TRK inhibitor
- **Brand Name:** Vitrakvi
- **Type Mechanism:** An orally available TRK inhibitor that binds to TRK, thereby preventing neurotrophin–TRK interaction and TRK activation, which results in both the induction of cellular apoptosis and the inhibition of cell growth in tumors that overexpress TRK
- **FDA Approval Date:** November 26, 2018
- **Indications:** Relapsed/refractory solid tumors, NHL, or histiocytic disorder with NTRK fusion
- **Dose:** 100 mg PO BID until PD
- **Half-life:** 3.5 hours
- **Side Effects:** Increased transaminases, fatigue, dizziness, anemia, dyspnea, neutropenia, constipation

(Hong et al., 2020; Laetsch et al., 2017)

Lasofoxifene

- **Manufacturer:** Sermonix

- **Type Mechanism:** Third-generation, selective estrogen receptor modulator, modifies the constitutive on confirmation of mutated ESR1 to antagonist confirmation, thereby inactivating the receptor
- **Drug Class:** Anti-estrogen
- **Trials:** Ongoing Phase 2 and 3 trials
- **Indications:** Metastatic breast cancer with *ESR1* mutations (FDA fast track designation for HR-positive MBC who harbor ESR1 mutations)
- **Dose:** 5 mg oral daily
- **Half-life:** ~7 days
- **Metabolism:** No significant CYP3A interaction
- **Side Effects:** Arthralgia, hot flashes, venous thromboembolism, visual disturbance

Lenvatinib Mesylate

- **Alias:** E7080
- **Type Mechanism:** A multitargeted TKI of VEGF receptors VEGFR1 (FLT1), VEGFR2 (KDR), VEGFR3 (FLT4), FGFR1, FGFR2, FGFR3, FGFR4, PDGFRα, KIT, and RET
- **FDA Approval Date:** February 13, 2015
- **Indications:** Differentiated thyroid carcinoma, advanced RCC, or endometrial cancer or unresectable HCC
- **Dose:** 18 mg daily (in combination with everolimus in the RCC); 24 mg daily (thyroid cancer); 20 mg daily in combination with pembrolizumab (endometrial cancer and RCC); 12 mg daily (HCC)
- **Half-life:** 28 hours
- **Metabolism:** Major CYP3A4 substrate
- **Side Effects:** HTN, proteinuria, nausea/vomiting, diarrhea, stomatitis, anorexia, fatigue, QT prolongation, peripheral edema, arthralgia, cough

LGK974

- **Alias:** KB-145911
- **Type Mechanism:** Small-molecule inhibitor of porcupine (PORCN) protein, important for Wnt pathway signaling. No published clinical results
- **Phase:** Ongoing phase 1 trial as single agent and in combination with anti–PD-1 in solid tumors
- **Dose:** 10 mg once daily
- **Half-life:** 5 to 8 hours
- **Side Effect:** Dysgeusia

(Liu et al., 2013; Rodon et al., 2021)

Lorlatinib

- **Alias:** Lorbrena

- **Type Mechanism:** Third-generation ALK inhibitor with increased potency and improved BBB penetration
- **FDA Approval Date:** November 2, 2018
- **Indications:** ALK-positive NSCLC
- **Dose:** 100 mg daily
- **Half-life:** 24 hours
- **Metabolism:** CY3A4 and UGT1A4
- **Side Effects:** HTN, edema, hyperlipidemia

(Shaw et al., 2017, 2019, 2020)

Lucitanib

- **Alias:** E-3810; AL3810
- **Type Mechanism:** Multikinase angiogenesis inhibitor of VEGFR1-3, PDGFRα/β, and FGFR1-3
- **Phase:** Phase 2/3 trial either alone and in combination with nivolumab for gynecologic cancers
- **Dose:** 6 mg PO once daily
- **Half-life:** 31 to 40 hours
- **Side Effects:** HTN, asthenia, proteinuria, rare thrombotic microangiopathy reported (two in phase 1 trial; one biopsy proven)

(Hui et al., 2020; Soria et al., 2015)

Lurbinectedin

- **Alias:** PM01183
- **Brand Name:** Zepzelca
- **Type Mechanism:** Alkylating agent that binds guanine residues in DNA, leading to cell-cycle disruption
- **FDA Approval Date:** June 15, 2020
- **Indications:** Metastatic SCLC
- **Dose:** 3.2 mg/m^2 IV Q 21 days
- **Half-life:** 51 hours
- **Metabolism:** Minor CYP3A4 substrate
- **Side Effects:** Cytopenias, hepatotoxicity, GI disorders
- **Clinical Pearls:** Body surface area (BSA) capped at 2 m^2 for dosing.

(Trigo et al., 2020)

Lutetium Lu 177 Dotatate

- **Brand Name:** Lutathera
- **Type Mechanism:** β- and γ-emitting radionuclide that binds to SSRT2. β Emission induces cellular damage by forming free radicals in somatostatin receptor–positive and surrounding cells.
- **Drug Class:** Radiopharmaceutical agent
- **FDA Approval Date:** January 26, 2018
- **Indications:** GEP-NETs
- **Dose:** 7.4 GBq (200 mCi) Q 7 weeks for 4 total doses
- **Half-life:** 71 ± 8 hours
- **Side Effects:** HTN, flushing, peripheral edema, alopecia, hyperglycemia,

hyperkalemia, GGT elevation, nausea, vomiting, abdominal pain, anemia, diarrhea, loss of appetite, leukopenia, lymphocytopenia, neutropenia, ALT/AST elevations, hyperbilirubinemia, fatigue
- **Clinical Pearls:** 68Ga-DOTATATE PET may help identify lesions and evaluate response.

(Strosberg et al., 2017)

Margetuximab-cmkb

- **Alias:** MGAH22
- **Brand Name:** Margenza
- **Type Mechanism:** A chimeric IgG1κ mAb antagonist against HER2. It exerts its effect by inhibiting HER2 shedding and through antibody-dependent cellular toxicity.
- **Drug Class:** Anti-HER2 mAb
- **FDA Approval Date:** December 16, 2020
- **Indications:** HER2-positive metastatic breast cancer
- **Dose:** 15 mg/kg IV Q 3 weeks in combination with chemotherapy
- **Half-life:** 19.2 days
- **Side Effects:** Hand-foot syndrome, reduction in LVEF, cytopenias
- **Clinical Pearls:** Anthracyclines may enhance the adverse/toxic effects and should be avoided for up to 4 months after discontinuing margetuximab.

Milademetan

- **Alias:** RAIN-32
- **Type Mechanism:** A small-molecule inhibitor of MDM2 that disrupts the interactions between MDM2 and the tumor suppressor protein p53. This will result in sustained increase in p53 activity with resultant antitumor effect.
- **Phase:** Phase 2; phase 3 in liposarcoma
- **Indications:** Well-differentiated/ dedifferentiated liposarcoma, intimal sarcoma, and advanced metastatic solid tumors with *MDM2* gene amplification
- **Dose:** RP2D: 260 mg PO daily on days 1 to 3 and days 15 to 17 of a 28-day cycle or 90 mg PO daily for 21 of 28 days
- **Metabolism:** Inhibitor of CYP3A4, P-glycoprotein, and BCRP
- **Side Effects:** Thrombocytopenia, neutropenia, anemia, nausea, decreased appetite, fatigue
- **Clinical Pearls:** Orphan drug designation for the treatment of liposarcoma.

(Takahashi et al., 2021)

Miransertib

- **Alias:** ARQ-092; MK-7075
- **Type Mechanism:** A small molecule that binds to and inhibits the activity of

AKT1/2/3 isoforms in a non–ATP-competitive manner, which may result in the inhibition of the PI3K/AKT signaling pathway. This may lead to the reduction in tumor cell proliferation and the induction of tumor cell apoptosis.

- **Phase:** Phase 1b
- **Indications:** PIK3CA or AKT1-mutant ER+ endometrial or ovarian cancer
- **Dose:** 150 mg PO daily for 5 days on, 9 days off (in combination with anastrozole)
- **Side Effects:** ALT elevation, rash, hyperglycemia

(Hyman et al., 2018)

Mirvetuximab Soravtansine

- **Alias:** IMGN853
- **Type Mechanism:** An immunoconjugate consisting of the humanized mAb M9346A against FOLR1 conjugated, via the disulfide-containing cleavable linker sulfo-PDB, to the cytotoxic maytansinoid DM4. After antibody–antigen interaction and internalization, the immunoconjugate releases DM4, which binds to tubulin and disrupts microtubule assembly/disassembly dynamics, thereby inhibiting cell division and the growth of FOLR1-expressing tumor cells.
- **Phase:** Phase 3 studies of mirvetuximab versus standard of care in advanced, epithelial ovarian cancer, primary peritoneal cancer, and/or fallopian tube cancer; phase 1/2 studies ongoing in combinations with chemotherapy, antiangiogenesis agents, and checkpoint inhibitors
- **Dose:** 6 mg/kg IV Q 3 weeks. Dose is based on actual ideal BW. May need to use prophylactic steroid eye drops to reduce ocular toxicities
- **Half-life:** 79 to 121 hours (3–5 days)
- **Side Effects:** Hypophosphatemia, keratitis, fatigue, diarrhea, infusion-related reactions, peripheral neuropathy

(Moore et al., 2017; O'Malley et al., 2020)

MK-0752

- **Type Mechanism:** A synthetic small-molecule γ-secretase that inhibits the Notch signaling pathway
- **Phase:** Phase 1/2
- **Indications:** T-cell leukemia, breast cancer, brain tumors (gliomas), pancreatic cancer, colon cancer, cervical cancer, and salivary gland carcinoma
- **Dose:** 350 mg PO 3 days on, 4 days off Q week for 28 days; 1,500 to 1,800 mg PO once a week with or without food

- **Half-life:** 15 hours (terminal)
- **Side Effects:** Nausea/vomiting, diarrhea, fatigue, lymphopenia, hypokalemia, constipation

(Krop et al., 2012)

MK-2206

- **Type Mechanism:** An allosteric inhibitor of AKT (protein kinase B)
- **Phase:** Phase 2
- **Indications:** Solid tumors
- **Dose:** 60 mg PO QOD on empty stomach, 2 hours before meal or 2 hours after meal
- **Half-life:** 63 to 89 hours
- **Metabolism:** Major CYP3A4 substrate
- **Side Effects:** Skin rash, stomatitis, nausea, pruritus, hyperglycemia, diarrhea

(Yap et al., 2011)

Napabucasin

- **Alias:** BBI608
- **Type Mechanism:** An orally available cancer cell stemness inhibitor that targets and inhibits multiple pathways involved in cancer cell stemness. This may ultimately inhibit cancer stemness cell (CSC) growth as well as heterogeneous cancer cell growth. It is also a small-molecule inhibitor of STAT3.
- **Phase:** Phase 3

- **Indications:** Advanced CRC, pancreatic cancer, GEJ cancer, gastric cancer
- **Dose:** 240 mg PO Q 12 hours
- **Half-life:** 1.5 to 2.7 hours
- **Metabolism:** Inhibitor of CYP1A2, CYP2B6, CYP2C8, CYP2C9, CYP2D6, and CYP3A4
- **Side Effects:** Diarrhea, anorexia, nausea, abdominal pain, fatigue, weight loss, dehydration
- **Clinical Pearls:** Orphan drug designation for gastric, GEJ, and pancreatic cancers in June 2016

(Jonker et al., 2018)

Navitoclax

- **Alias:** ABT-263
- **Type Mechanism:** An orally potent and highly selective inhibitor of antiapoptotic members of the BCL-2 family, with a nanomolar affinity for BCL-2, BCL-xL, and BCL-w
- **Phase:** Phase 3 studies in myelofibrosis; phase 1/2 studies in advanced solid tumors
- **Dose:** Up to 250 mg PO daily on a 21-day cycle
- **Half-life:** 15 hours
- **Side Effects:** Nausea/vomiting/diarrhea, fatigue/dizziness, thrombocytopenia, neutropenia, pyrexia, increased ALT

(Gandhi et al., 2011)

Necitumumab

- **Alias:** IMC-11F8
- **Type Mechanism:** A recombinant human IgG1 EGFR mAb that binds (with a high affinity) to the ligand-binding site of the EGFR to prevent receptor activation and downstream signaling
- **FDA Approval Date:** November 24, 2015
- **Indications:** FDA approved for metastatic SCC of the lungs (NSCLC)
- **Dose:** 800 mg IV over 60 minutes on days 1 and 8 of a 3-week cycle in combination with gemcitabine/cisplatin until PD
- **Half-life:** 14 days
- **Side Effects:** Headache, rash (acneiform eruption), electrolyte imbalance (potassium, phosphorus, calcium, magnesium), diarrhea, vomiting, stomatitis

Neratinib

- **Alias:** HKI-272; PB272
- **Type Mechanism:** Irreversible pan-EGFR inhibitor that can potentially overcome the acquired resistance of EGFR T790M mutation by targeting a cysteine residue in the ATP-binding pocket of the receptor
- **FDA Approval Date:** July 17, 2017
- **Indications:** FDA approved for extended adjuvant therapy in HER2-positive breast cancer; for the treatment of adult patients with advanced or metastatic HER2-positive breast cancer who have received two or more prior anti-HER2-based regimens in the metastatic setting (in combination with capecitabine)
- **Dose:** 240 mg PO daily with food
- **Half-life:** 14 hours (range 7–17 hours)
- **Side Effects:** Diarrhea, nausea/vomiting, fatigue, anorexia, skin rash, stomatitis
- **Clinical Pearls:** Recommend to use antidiarrheal prophylaxis with loperamide.

Nintedanib

- **Alias:** BIBF1120
- **Brand Name:** Ofev (the United States); Vargatef (European Union)
- **Type Mechanism:** A triple angiokinase inhibitor of VEGFR1, VEGFR2, VEGFR3, PDGFRα, PDGFRβ, FGFR1, FGFR2, FGFR3
- **FDA Approval Date:** October 15, 2014
- **Indications:** Approved in combination with docetaxel in EU for NSCLC after first-line therapy. FDA approved for chronic fibrosing interstitial lung disease and idiopathic pulmonary fibrosis
- **Dose:** 150 mg BID in lung diseases

- **Half-life:** 9.5 hours
- **Side Effects:** Diarrhea, nausea/vomiting, anorexia, liver dysfunction (hyperbilirubinemia, transaminitis), increased amylase/lipase, HTN

(Gandhi et al., 2011; Richeldi et al., 2014)

Niraparib

- **Alias:** MK-4827
- **Brand Name:** Zejula
- **Type Mechanism:** An inhibitor of PARP-1 and PARP-2
- **FDA Approval Date:** March 27, 2017
- **Indications:** FDA approved for recurrent epithelial ovarian cancer, fallopian tube or primary peritoneal cancer patients who are in CR or partial response (PR) to platinum-based chemotherapy
- **Dose:** 300 mg PO daily with or without food
- **Half-life:** 36 hours (range 33–46 hours)
- **Metabolism:** CYP1A2 and CYP3A4; P-glycoprotein
- **Side Effects:** Fatigue, insomnia, pneumonitis, anorexia, constipation, nausea/vomiting, neutropenia, thrombocytopenia

---

Nirogacestat

- **Alias:** PF-03084014

- **Type Mechanism:** An oral small-molecule γ-secretase inhibitor
- **Phase:** FDA granted orphan drug designation for desmoid tumors and European Commission for STSs
- **Dose:** 150 mg BID (changed from prior version)
- **Half-life:** 22 to 40 hours
- **Side Effects:** Diarrhea, nausea, fatigue, hypophosphatemia, vomiting

(Messersmith et al., 2015)

Nivolumab

- **Alias:** BMS-936558; MDX1106; ONO-4538
- **Brand Name:** Opdivo
- **Type Mechanism:** Fully human IgG4 mAb targeting PD-1 receptor on activated T cells
- **FDA Approval Date:** December 22, 2014
- **Indications:** FDA approved for recurrent or metastatic SCCHN, classic Hodgkin lymphoma, unresectable or metastatic melanoma or in adjuvant setting, metastatic NSCLC (nonsquamous), advanced RCC, RCC, HCC, MSI-H CRC, and locally advanced or metastatic urothelial carcinoma
- **Dose:** 3 mg/kg IV Q 2 weeks (H&N cancer, Hodgkin lymphoma, SCLC); 240 mg IV Q 2 weeks or 480 mg IV Q 4 weeks (melanoma,

NSCLC, RCC, urothelial cancer, MSI-H CRC, esophageal cancer, HCC); mesothelioma 360 mg IV Q 3 weeks in combination with ipilimumab; combination and then increase it to 3 mg/kg or 240 mg when given alone (HCC, melanoma, RCC)

- **Half-life:** 25 days
- **Side Effects:** Fatigue, nausea, diarrhea, xerostomia, pruritus, immune-mediated colitis, pneumonitis, hyperglycemia, hypertriglyceridemia, hyponatremia, thyroid dysfunction

Obatoclax Mesylate

- **Alias:** GX15-070
- **Type Mechanism:** A small molecule and a pan inhibitor of Bcl-2 family proteins, with proapoptotic activity. GX015-070 is a selective antagonist of the BH3-binding groove of the Bcl-2 family proteins, which are frequently overexpressed in cancers, including CLL. This agent induces/restores apoptosis in cancer cells by inhibiting apoptosis suppressors in multiple members of the Bcl-2 family simultaneously.
- **Drug Class:** Pan-bcl-2 inhibitor
- **Phase:** Phase 2
- **Indications:** SCLC, MDSs, relapsed/refractory MCL
- **Dose:** 60 mg IV over 24 hours Q 2 weeks
- **Side Effects:** Euphoria, nausea, diarrhea, anemia, ataxia, thrombocytopenia, pneumonia
- **Clinical Pearls:** Phase 2 with topotecan for relapsed SCLC did not show superiority over historic response rate with topotecan alone.

(Paik et al., 2011)

Olaparib

- **Alias:** AZD2281; KU-0059436
- **Brand Name:** Lynparza
- **Type Mechanism:** A small-molecule inhibitor of the nuclear enzyme PARP with potential chemosensitizing and radiosensitizing properties
- **FDA Approval Date:** December 19, 2014
- **Indications:** Advanced ovarian cancer, HER2-negative and BRCA mutation breast cancer, MCRPC with HRD, and pancreatic cancer as maintenance therapy after first-line chemotherapy
- **Dose:** 400 mg Q 12 hours. No grapefruit or Seville oranges
- **Half-life:** 11.9 ± 4.8 hours

- **Side Effects:** Nausea/vomiting, leukopenia/lymphopenia, increased creatinine, fatigue, abdominal pain, diarrhea, anemia, thrombocytopenia, muscle pain, infection

Onartuzumab

- **Alias:** MetMAb; RO5490258
- **Type Mechanism:** An IgG1 humanized monovalent mAb that is directed against MET by binding to the extracellular domain, preventing the binding of its ligand, HGF
- **Phase:** Phase 3
- **Indications:** NSCLC and MET+ GE cancer
- **Dose:** 15 mg/kg IV Q 3 weeks
- **Half-life:** 8 to 12 days
- **Side Effects:** Fatigue, peripheral edema, nausea, hypoalbuminemia

(Salgia et al., 2014)

Onatasertib

- **Alias:** CC-223
- **Type Mechanism:** A potent, selective, and orally bioavailable inhibitor of mTOR kinase, demonstrating inhibition of mTORC1 (pS6RP and p4EBP1) and mTORC2 [pAKT(S473)] in cellular systems. mTOR kinase inhibition in cells, by CC-223, resulted in more complete inhibition of the mTOR pathway biomarkers and improved antiproliferative activity as compared with rapamycin.
- **Drug Class:** mTOR inhibitor
- **Phase:** Phase 2
- **Indications:** Non-pNETs, MM, and NHL
- **Dose:** 30 mg PO daily for 28 days
- **Half-life:** 4.86 to 5.64 hours
- **Side Effects:** Diarrhea, fatigue, stomatitis, hyperglycemia, rash, thrombocytopenia, decreased appetite, transaminitis

(Mortensen et al., 2015)

Palbociclib

- **Alias:** PD0332991
- **Brand Name:** Ibrance
- **Type Mechanism:** A reversible small-molecule CDK inhibitor that is selective for CDK 4 and CDK 6. CDKs have a role in regulating progression through the cell cycle at the G1/S phase by blocking Rb hyperphosphorylation. It reduces the proliferation of breast cancer cell lines by preventing progression from the G1 to the S cell-cycle phase.
- **FDA Approval Date:** February 3, 2015

- **Indications:** FDA approved with hormone therapy for HR-positive, HER2-negative breast cancer or advanced breast cancer as initial endocrine-based therapy or upon PD with endocrine therapy
- **Dose:** 125 mg PO daily for 21 days of the 28-day cycle. No grapefruit juice
- **Half-life:** 29 ± 5 hours
- **Metabolism:** Major CYP3A4 substrate
- **Side Effects:** Fatigue, nausea/vomiting, diarrhea, constipation, rash, peripheral edema, dyspnea, myelosuppression, stomatitis

(Finn et al., 2016)

Panitumumab

- **Alias:** ABX-EGF; mAb ABX-EGF; rHuMAb-EGFr
- **Brand Name:** Vectibix
- **Type Mechanism:** A fully human mAb that binds specifically to EGFR on both normal and tumor cells and competitively inhibits the binding of ligands for EGFR
  - First antibody to demonstrate the use of KRAS as a predictive biomarker
- **FDA Approval Date:** September 27, 2006
- **Indications:** FDA approved for RAS WT mCRC
- **Dose:** 6 mg/kg IV infusion (over 60 or 90 minutes) Q 14 days

- **Half-life:** 7.5 days (range 4–11 days)
- **Side Effects:** Dermatologic toxicity (rash, dermatitis acneiform, pruritus) (U.S. box warning), infusion reactions (fevers, chills, bronchospasms) (U.S. box warning), hypomagnesemia, paronychia, fatigue, nausea/vomiting, diarrhea
- **Clinical Pearls:** Severity of acne-form rash can be minimized with the use of topical steroid cream, topical antibiotic gel, and doxycycline. Presence and severity of rash may correlate improved response and survival.

(Peeters et al., 2009)

Pazopanib Hydrochloride

- **Alias:** GW786034
- **Brand Name:** Votrient
- **Type Mechanism:** Selectively inhibits VEGFR1, VEGFR2, VEGFR3, FGFR1, FGFR3, KIT, and PDGFR, preventing angiogenesis
- **FDA Approval Date:** October 19, 2009
- **Indications:** FDA approved for RCC and STS
- **Dose:** 800 mg daily on fasting stomach, at least 1 hour before or 2 hours after a meal; avoid grapefruit juice
- **Half-life:** 31 hours
- **Metabolism:** Major CYP3A4 substrate

- **Side Effects:** Diarrhea, nausea/vomiting, anorexia, HTN, hair color changes (lightening)
- **Clinical Pearls:** Avoid concurrent medications, which can prolong the QTc interval. Because VEGFR is inhibited, surgical intervention should be avoided.

Pembrolizumab

- **Alias:** MK-3475; SCH 900475
- **Brand Name:** Keytruda
- **Type Mechanism:** A humanized IgG4 mAb directed against human cell-surface receptor PD-1, an inhibitory signaling receptor expressed on the surface of activated T cells. This results in the activation of T-cell–mediated immune responses against tumor cells.
- **FDA Approval Date:** September 4, 2014; November 13, 2020 (locally recurrent unresectable or metastatic TNBC whose tumors express PD-L1 (CPS ≥10), in combination with chemotherapy); July 26, 2021 (high-risk early-stage TNBC, in combination with chemotherapy)
- **Indications:** FDA approved for recurrent or metastatic SCCHN, adult and pediatric patients with relapsed or refractory Hodgkin lymphoma, unresectable or metastatic melanoma, adjuvant therapy for melanoma, unresectable or metastatic MSI-H cancers, metastatic NSCLC with PD-L1 expression, or locally advanced or metastatic urothelial carcinoma; for the treatment of patients with locally recurrent unresectable or metastatic triple-negative breast cancer (TNBC) whose tumors express PD-L1 (CPS ≥10) as determined by an FDA-approved test, in combination with chemotherapy; high-risk, early-stage TNBC in combination with chemotherapy as neoadjuvant treatment, and then continued as a single agent as adjuvant treatment after surgery.
- **Dose:** 200 mg IV Q 3 weeks or 400 mg IV Q 6 weeks
- **Side Effects:** Fatigue, rash, hyperglycemia, hypertriglyceridemia, hyponatremia, diarrhea, decreased appetite, anemia, muscle pain, increased SCr, infection, thyroid disorder, immune-mediated pneumonitis

---

Pemigatinib

- **Brand Name:** Pemazyre
- **Type Mechanism:** Oral competitive inhibitor of FGFR1-3 inhibiting FGFR phosphorylation
- **FDA Approval Date:** April 17, 2020

- **Indications:** FDA approved for locally advanced, unresectable, or metastatic cholangiocarcinoma with FGFR2 alteration
- **Dose:** 13.5 mg once daily on days 1 to 14 of a 21-day cycle
- **Half-life:** 15.4 hours
- **Metabolism:** Primarily hepatic through CYP3A4
- **Side Effects:** Edema, hyperphosphatemia, ocular toxicity (retinal pigment epithelial detachment)

(Abou-Alfa et al., 2020)

Peposertib

- **Alias:** Nedisertib; MSC2490484A; M3814
- **Type Mechanism:** A small-molecule, selective DNA-PK inhibitor that blocks DNA-PK activity inhibiting its ability to function in the DNA repair process. This leads to DNA DSB persistence and subsequent cellular death.
- **Phase:** Phase 1 in combination with RT and/or chemotherapy
- **Dose:** 400 mg BID
- **Half-life:** ~5.5 hours
- **Side Effects:** Nausea/vomiting, fatigue, rash, pyrexia

(van Bussel et al., 2021)

Pertuzumab

- **Alias:** 2C4; rhuMAb-2C4
- **Type Mechanism:** A humanized recombinant mAb directed against the extracellular dimerization domain of the HER2
- **FDA Approval Date:** June 8, 2012
- **Indications:** FDA approved for HER2-positive breast cancer
- **Dose:** A loading dose of 840 mg IV infusion (over 60 minutes); a maintenance dose of 420 mg IV infusion (over 30–60 minutes) Q 3 weeks; approved to be given in combination with trastuzumab and docetaxel
- **Half-life:** 18 days
- **Side Effects:** Diarrhea, fatigue, neutropenia, rash, nausea/vomiting, stomatitis, embryo–fetal toxicity/cardiotoxicity (U.S. box warning)

Pilaralisib

- **Alias:** SAR245408; XL-147
- **Type Mechanism:** An orally bioavailable small molecule targeting the class I PI3K family
- **Phase:** No ongoing trials registered
- **Indications:** Currently in phase 2 trial for endometrial cancers, phase 1b/2 trial for HR-positive breast cancer
- **Dose:** 600 mg PO daily as continuous dosing
- **Half-life:** 70 to 88 hours

- **Side Effects:** Maculopapular rash, nausea, diarrhea, decreased appetite

(Matulonis et al., 2015)

Pimasertib

- **Alias:** MSC1936369B; AS703026
- **Type Mechanism:** Selective noncompetitive ATP inhibitor of MEK1/2
- **Phase:** Phase 1/2
- **Dose:** 60 mg PO daily
- **Side Effects:** Diarrhea, CPK increase
- **Clinical Pearls:** Crosses BBB

(Awada et al., 2012; Lebbé et al., 2020)

Ponatinib Hydrochloride

- **Alias:** AP24534
- **Brand Name:** Iclusig
- **Type Mechanism:** A multitargeted RTK inhibitor of WT and all mutated forms of BCR-ABL, including T315I, the highly drug therapy–resistant missense mutation of BCR-ABL
  - Also inhibits VEGFR, FGFR, TIE2, and FLT3
- **FDA Approval Date:** December 14, 2012
- **Indications:** Chronic myeloid leukemia with T315I-positive mutation in chronic, accelerated, or blastic phase or have resistance or intolerance to at least two prior kinase inhibitors. Also indicated for acute lymphoblastic leukemia with Philadelphia chromosome-positive (Ph+) for which no other kinase inhibitors are indicated or ALL Ph+ with T315I mutation positive.
- **Dose:** 45 mg PO with or without food
- **Half-life:** 24 hours
- **Metabolism:** Moderate CYP3A4 substrate
- **Side Effects:** HTN, peripheral edema, rash, nausea/vomiting, abdominal pain, myelosuppression, fatigue/weakness, diarrhea or constipation, increased lipase, hyperglycemia, arterial thrombosis/ hepatotoxicity (U.S. box warning)

Poziotinib

- **Alias:** HM781-36B; NOV120101; pan-HER kinase inhibitor HM781-36B
- **Type Mechanism:** A quinazoline-based, small molecular and irreversible inhibitor of EGFR (HER1 or ErbB1), ceritinib HER2, HER4, and EGFR mutants with exon 20 insertion
- **Phase:** Phase 2
- **Indications:** EGFR-mutated advanced NSCLC with exon 20 insertion mutations, HER2-positive metastatic breast cancer patients who have received two prior lines

of HER2 therapies, and in HER2-positive gastric cancer patients
- **Dose:** 12 to 16 mg PO daily for 14 days on, 7 days off in a fasted state
- **Half-life:** 5.1 to 9.9 hours on day 1 and similar on day 14
- **Side Effects:** Diarrhea, rash, fatigue, pruritus, stomatitis, anorexia

(Kim et al., 2018; Park et al., 2018)

Pralsetinib

- **Alias:** BLU-667
- **Brand Name:** Gavreto
- **Type Mechanism:** A next-generation small-molecule RET inhibitor designed to target oncogenic RET fusions and mutations
- **Phase:** Phase 3
- **FDA Approval Date:** September 4, 2020
- **Indications:** Accelerated FDA approval for RET fusion–positive NSCLC and RET fusion or mutation-positive thyroid cancer
- **Dose:** 400 mg PO once daily
- **Half-life:** 16 hours after single dose, 20 hours after multiple doses
- **Metabolism:** Major CYP3A4 substrate
- **Side Effects:** Increased AST/ALT, cytopenias, fatigue, HTN, hypophosphatemia

(Subbiah et al., 2020)

Prexasertib

- **Alias:** LY2606368
- **Type Mechanism:** An ATP-competitive inhibitor of CHK1 and CHK2 that selectively binds CHK1 to prevent DNA damage repair
- **Phase:** Phase 1/2 trials
- **Dose:** 105 mg/m^2 IV Q 14 days in a 28-day cycle
- **Half-life:** 13 to 27 hours
- **Side Effects:** Cytopenias with risk for febrile neutropenia

(Hong et al., 2019; Lee et al., 2018)

Pyrotinib

- **Type Mechanism:** An orally irreversible pan-ErbB receptor tyrosine kinase inhibitor that targets HER1, HER2, and HER4
- **Indications:** Approved in China and used in combination with capecitabine for HER2-positive, advanced metastatic breast cancer following anthracycline or taxane
- **Dose:** 400 mg PO once daily
- **Half-life:** 11.4 to 15.9 hours
- **Metabolism:** CYP3A4 most active enzyme, primarily excreted through feces
- **Side Effects:** Diarrhea, hand-foot syndrome, vomiting

(Ma et al., 2019; Xu et al., 2021)

Ramucirumab

- **Alias:** IMC-1121B
- **Brand Name:** Cyramza
- **Type Mechanism:** A recombinant, fully human mAb directed against VEGFR2. Has a high affinity for VEGFR2, binding to it and blocking the binding of VEGFR ligands VEGF-A, VEGF-C, and VEGF-D to inhibit the activation of VEGFR2, thereby inhibiting ligand-induced proliferation and migration of endothelial cells. VEGFR2 inhibition results in reduced tumor vascularity and growth.
- **FDA Approval Date:** April 21, 2014
- **Indications:** FDA approved for mCRC, advanced or metastatic gastric cancer, metastatic NSCLC, HCC
- **Dose:** 8 mg/kg IV Q 2 weeks (CRC and gastric cancer); 10 mg/kg IV Q 21 days (NSCLC)
- **Half-life:** 14 days
- **Side Effects:** Nausea/vomiting, headache, fatigue, proteinuria, HTN, abdominal pain, DVT

(Tabernero et al., 2015; Wilke et al., 2014)

RC48-ADC

- **Type Mechanism:** A novel humanized anti-HER2 antibody conjugated with a cleavable linker to MMAE

- **Phase:** Phase 1/2
- **Dose:** 2.0 mg/kg IV over 30 to 90 minutes Q 2 weeks
- **Half-life:** 1 to 1.5 days
- **Side Effects:** AST/ALT increase, hypoesthesia, cytopenias

(Sheng et al., 2021)

Rebastinib

- **Alias:** DCC-2036
- **Type Mechanism:** Switch-control inhibitor targeting tunica interna endothelial cell kinase (Tie-2)
- **Phase:** Phase 1/2
- **Dose:** 50 mg BID PO in combination with paclitaxel
- **Half-life:** 12 to 15 hours
- **Side Effects:** Constipation, fatigue, alopecia, peripheral edema, dysgeusia, peripheral neuropathy, diarrhea, arthralgia

(Janku et al., 2020)

Refametinib

- **Alias:** BAY 86-9766; RDEA119
- **Type Mechanism:** Highly selective, orally bioavailable inhibitor of MEK 1/2
- **Phase:** Phase 1/2

- **Indications:** Highly selective, orally bioavailable inhibitor of MEK 1/2
- **Dose:** 100 mg PO daily
- **Half-life:** 12 hours
- **Metabolism:** Substrates of CYP3A4 and CYP2C19; concomitant use of inhibitors or inducers of these enzymes should be avoided.
- **Side Effects:** Acneiform dermatitis, diarrhea, nausea/vomiting, lymphedema, fatigue, rash

(Weekes et al., 2013)

Regorafenib

- **Alias:** BAY 73-4506
- **Type Mechanism:** Orally bioavailable VEGFR, TIE2, KIT, RAF, RET, PDGFR, FGFR inhibitor
- **FDA Approval Date:** September 27, 2012
- **Indications:** FDA approved for mCRC and unresectable or metastatic GISTs and HCC
- **Dose:** 160 mg PO with food, once daily for the first 21 days of each 28-day cycle
- **Half-life:** 28 hours (range 14–58 hours)
- **Metabolism:** Major CYP3A4 substrate
- **Side Effects:** Hepatotoxicity (U.S. box warning), asthenia/fatigue, diarrhea, anorexia, HTN, mucositis, dysphonia
- **Clinical Pearls:** Assure liver function tests before initiation; monitor blood pressure closely; for diarrhea, prescribe imodium— up to 8 tabs/day. If resistant, first add budesonide 3-mg tab TID, and possibly also add third drug, lomotil, 2 tab four times daily (QID). For mucositis, avoid sodas, acidic fruits, tomatoes, and spicy food. Gargle with baking soda/water mixture am/pm and after each meal. Swish with carafate after baking soda to coat the mouth and protect. May also add viscous lidocaine to assist with diminishing painful eating. For anorexia, add supplemental nutrition to each meal: ensure/ boost TID if feasible.

Ribociclib

- **Alias:** LEE011
- **Brand Name:** Kisqali
- **Type Mechanism:** A reversible small-molecule CDK inhibitor that is selective for CDK4 and 6. CDKs have a role in regulating progression through the cell cycle at the G1/S phase by blocking retinoblastoma (Rb) hyperphosphorylation. It reduces the proliferation of breast cancer cell lines by preventing progression from the G1 to the S cell-cycle phase.
- **FDA Approval Date:** March 13, 2017
- **Indications (1):** FDA approved with hormone therapy for hormone

receptor–positive, HER2-negative breast cancer or advanced breast cancer as initial endocrine-based therapy or upon disease progression with endocrine therapy
- **Dose:** 600 mg PO daily for 21 days of the 28-day cycle. No grapefruit juice
- **Half-life:** Mean 32 hours (29.7 to 54.7 hours)
- **Metabolism:** Major CYP3A4 substrate
- **Side Effects:** Fatigue, nausea/vomiting, diarrhea, alopecia, constipation, rash, peripheral edema, dyspnea, myelosuppression, stomatitis, QT prolongation, pneumonitis

Ripretinib

- **Brand Name:** Qinlock
- **Type Mechanism:** A switch-control TKI active against a broad spectrum of KIT and PDGFRα mutations through binding to WT and mutant forms, preventing switch from inactive to active conformations
- **Phase:** Phase 3
- **Indications:** FDA approved the fourth-line treatment of GIST
- **Dose:** 150 mg daily
- **Half-life:** 14.8 hours
- **Side Effects:** Increased lipase, HTN, hypophosphatemia, diarrhea, anemia

(Blay et al., 2020)

Rucaparib Camsylate

- **Alias:** AG014699; CO-338; PF-01367338
- **Brand Name:** Rubraca
- **Type Mechanism:** The camsylate salt form of rucaparib, an inhibitor of the nuclear enzyme polyadenosine 5′-diphosphoribose PARP, with chemosensitizing, radiosensitizing, and antineoplastic activities. Rucaparib selectively binds to PARP-1, PARP-2, and PARP-3 and inhibits PARP-1-mediated repair of single-strand DNA (ssDNA) breaks via the base-excision repair pathway. This enhances the accumulation of DNA strand breaks and promotes genomic instability and apoptosis. Rucaparib may potentiate the cytotoxicity of DNA-damaging agents and reverse tumor cell resistance to chemotherapy and RT.
- **FDA Approval Date:** December 19, 2016
- **Indications:** FDA approved as monotherapy for the treatment of patients with deleterious BRCA mutation (germline or somatic) associated with advanced ovarian cancer in advanced or recurrent setting (as maintenance) and approved for BRCA-mutated MCRPC
- **Dose:** 600 mg BID
- **Half-life:** 17 to 19 hours

- **Side Effects:** Fatigue, increased cholesterol, nausea/vomiting, constipation, decreased appetite, dysgeusia, abdominal pain, thrombocytopenia, anemia, transaminitis, weakness, increased SCr, photosensitivity

(Abida et al., 2020; Jenner et al., 2016)

Ruxolitinib Phosphate

- **Alias:** INCB18424; Jakavi (Canada)
- **Brand Name:** Jakafi
- **Type Mechanism:** An oral kinase inhibitor that inhibits JAK1 and JAK2
- **FDA Approval Date:** November 16, 2011
- **Indications:** FDA approved for intermediate- or high-risk myelofibrosis, GvHD, and polycythemia vera (PV)
- **Dose:** Platelets $\geq$200,000/mm^3, start 20 mg PO BID; platelets $\geq$100,000/mm^3, start 15 mg PO BID; platelets $\geq$50,000/mm^3, start 5 mg PO BID; may titrate all doses in increments of 5 mg PO BID Q 2 weeks to maximum dose of 25 mg PO BID with or without food (myelofibrosis); 10 mg PO BID (GvHD and PV)
- **Half-life:** 5.8 hours
- **Metabolism:** Potent CYP3A4 substrate
- **Side Effects:** Diarrhea, peripheral edema, dizziness/headache, increased ALT/AST, myelosuppression (thrombocytopenia, neutropenia, anemia), ecchymosis

Sacituzumab Govitecan

- **Brand Name:** Trodelvy
- **Type Mechanism:** An ADC with a humanized TROP2 antibody with a topoisomerase inhibitor SN-38 payload via a cleavable linker
- **FDA Approval Date:** April 22, 2020
- **Indications:** Approved for advanced, refractory, or metastatic TNBC after two or more treatments and locally advanced or metastatic urothelial cancer after platinum and checkpoint inhibitor
- **Dose:** 10 mg/kg IV on days 1 and 8 of a 21-day cycle
- **Half-life:** 15.3 hours
- **Metabolism:** SN38 primarily metabolized via UGT1A1
- **Side Effects:** Cytopenias including neutropenia, diarrhea, hypersensitivity, neuropathy

(Bardia et al., 2019; Tagawa et al., 2021)

Sapanisertib

- **Alias:** TAK228; MLN0128; INK128
- **Type Mechanism:** An orally bioavailable mTOR1/2 inhibitor
- **Phase:** Ongoing phase 1 trials either alone and in combination
- **Dose:** 5 mg daily or 30 mg weekly

- **Half-life:** 5.9 to 9.4 hours
- **Side Effects:** Hyperglycemia, rash, stomatitis, asthenia

(Voss et al., 2020)

Selinexor

- **Alias:** KPT-330
- **Type Mechanism:** A small-molecule inhibitor of CRM1 (chromosome region maintenance 1 protein, exportin 1 or XPO1), with potential antineoplastic activity
  - Modifies the essential CRM1 cargo–binding residue cysteine-528, thereby irreversibly inactivating CRM1-mediated nuclear export of cargo proteins such as tumor suppressor proteins, including p53, p21, BRCA1/2, pRB, FOXO, and other growth regulatory proteins
  - Restores endogenous tumor suppressing processes to selectively eliminate tumor cells, while sparing normal cells
- **FDA Approval Date:** July 3, 2019
- **Indications:** Approved in relapsed or refractory DLBCL and MM
- **Dose:** DLBCL: 60 mg/dose on days 1 and 3 each week; MM Sd regimen: 80 mg/dose on days 1 and 3 each week; MM SVd regimen: 100 mg once weekly on day 1
- **Half-life:** 6 to 7 hours

- **Side Effects:** Anorexia, asthenia, cytopenias, edema, fatigue, hyponatremia, liver function elevations

(Abdul Razak et al., 2016)

Selitrectinib

- **Alias:** LOXO-195
- **Type Mechanism:** Selective second-generation TRK inhibitor to maintain potency against multiple TRK domain mutations
- **Phase:** Phase 1/2
- **Half-life:** 3 hours
- **Side Effects:** Dizziness/ataxia, gait disturbance, nausea/vomiting, anemia, thrombocytopenia, myalgia, abdominal pain

(Hyman et al., 2019)

Selpercatinib

- **Alias:** LOXO-292
- **Brand Name:** Retevmo
- **Type Mechanism:** An ATP-competitive selective small-molecule RET kinase inhibitor
- **Drug Class:** RET inhibitor
- **FDA Approval Date:** May 8, 2020
- **Indications:** RET fusion–positive NSCLC or thyroid cancer or RET-mutant MTC

- **Dose:** >50 kg: 160 mg BID; <50 kg: 120 mg BID
- **Half-life:** 32 hours
- **Metabolism:** Predominantly CYP3A4
- **Side Effects:** Dry mouth, fatigue, HTN

(Wirth et al., 2020)

Selumetinib

- **Alias:** AZD6244; ARRY-142886
- **Brand Name:** Koselugo
- **Type Mechanism:** An orally bioavailable small molecule that inhibits MEK or MAPK/ERKs 1 and 2
- **Phase:** Phase 3
- **Indications:** FDA approved for neurofibromatosis type 1 with symptomatic, inoperable plexiform neurofibromas
- **Dose:** 50 to 75 mg PO BID
- **Half-life:** 8.3 hours
- **Side Effects:** Nausea/vomiting, weight gain, acneiform dermatitis, diarrhea, peripheral edema

(Gross et al., 2020)

Serabelisib

- **Alias:** TAK-117; INK-1117; MLN-1117
- **Type Mechanism:** A selective oral PI3Kα isoform inhibitor demonstrating greater selectivity than other class I PI3K family members and mTOR, and a high degree of selectivity against many other kinases
- **Phase:** Ongoing phase 1–2 studies
- **Dose:** TIW of 900 mg daily oral (e.g., MWF/MTuW) or 150 mg PO oral daily
- **Half-life:** ~11 hours
- **Side Effects:** Nausea, hyperglycemia, hyperglycemia, elevated liver transaminases

(Juric et al., 2017)

Sintilimab

- **Brand Name:** Tyvyt
- **Type Mechanism:** Fully human IgG4 mAb that targets checkpoint inhibitor PD-1 and blocks its interaction with PD-L1 and PD-L2; this results in releasing the PD-1 pathway–mediated inhibition of the immune response, including antitumor immune response, thereby decreasing tumor growth
- **Phase:** Phase 3 pending FDA approval
- **Indications:** FDA accepted for review the Biologics License Application (BLA) for sintilimab in combination with pemetrexed and platinum chemotherapy for the first-line treatment of nonsquamous NSCLC chemotherapy
- **Dose:** 200 mg IV Q 3 weeks
- **Half-life:** 35.6 hours

- **Side Effects:** Hypothyroidism, rash, diarrhea, increased liver function tests, pruritis

(Yang et al., 2020)

Sonolisib

- **Alias:** PX-866; CHEBI:65345; DJM-166
- **Type Mechanism:** An irreversible, small-molecule wortmannin analog inhibitor of the α, γ, and δ isoforms of PI3K
- **Phase:** Phase 1/2
- **Indications:** CRC, melanoma, glioblastoma multiforme, SCCHN, and prostate cancer
- **Dose:** 8 mg PO daily on fasting stomach 2 hours before meals and fast for 1 hour after dosing
- **Half-life:** 4 hours
- **Side Effects:** Nausea/vomiting, diarrhea, fatigue, thrombocytopenia, increased AST

(Hong et al., 2012)

Sorafenib

- **Alias:** BAY 43-9006
- **Brand Name:** Nexavar
- **Type Mechanism:** Orally bioavailable inhibitor of RAF, VEGFR, PDGFRβ, and RET
- **FDA Approval Date:** December 20, 2005
- **Indications:** FDA approved for RCC, HCC, and differentiated thyroid carcinoma

- **Dose:** 400 mg PO BID without food (at least 1 hour before or 2 hours after a meal)
- **Half-life:** 25 to 48 hours
- **Metabolism:** UGT1A1 inhibitor; a weak substrate of CYP3A4
- **Side Effects:** Rash, redness, itching, or peeling of skin; alopecia; diarrhea; nausea/vomiting; anorexia; abdominal pain; fatigue
- **Clinical Pearls:** Avoid direct sunlight, use moisturizers after therapy, use mild soap for bathing, and antihistamine for itching. Monitor the patient's blood pressure while on therapy. Instruct the patient on home monitoring. Monitor PTT/INR (International normalized ratio) closely for patients taking Coumadin.

Sotorasib

- **Alias:** AMG510
- **Brand Name:** Lumakras
- **Type Mechanism:** A small molecule that specifically and irreversibly inhibits KRAS G12C through interaction at the P2 pocket, trapping it in the inactive GDP-bound state
- **Phase:** Ongoing phase 3 studies
- **Indications:** Approved in locally advanced or metastatic KRAS G12C-mutated NSCLC
- **Dose:** 960 mg PO once daily

- **Half-life:** 5 hours
- **Metabolism:** CYP3A4 substrate and moderate inducer of CYP3A4
- **Side Effects:** Diarrhea, cytopenias, hepatotoxicity, fatigue, edema, hyponatremia, rash

(Hong et al., 2020; Skoulidis et al., 2021)

Spartalizumab

- **Alias:** PDR001
- **Type Mechanism:** A humanized checkpoint inhibitors mAb directed toward PD-1.
- **Phase:** Ongoing phase 1–3 studies
- **Dose:** 400 mg Q 4 weeks or 300 mg Q 3 weeks
- **Half-life:** 11 to 41 days
- **Side Effects:** Fatigue, diarrhea, hypothyroidism, hyponatremia, transaminase elevation

(Naing et al., 2020)

Sunitinib

- **Alias:** SU11248
- **Type Mechanism:** Antiangiogenesis inhibitor of PDGFR and VEGFR, as well as KIT and RET
- **FDA Approval Date:** January 26, 2006
- **Indications:** FDA approved in GIST, pNET, and RCC

- **Dose:** 50 mg daily, 4 weeks on treatment followed by 2 weeks off. pNET dose: 37.5 mg daily, continuously without a scheduled off-treatment period
- **Half-life:** 40 to 60 hours
- **Side Effects:** Hepatotoxicity (U.S. box warning), yellowing of skin, fatigue, pyrexia, diarrhea, nausea/vomiting, rash
- **Clinical Pearls:** Swelling of the face, upper, and lower extremities is a possible side effect. Higher risk of complications such as osteonecrosis when taking bisphosphonates with this drug is also possible.

Talazoparib Tosylate

- **Alias:** BMN-673
- **Type Mechanism:** A potent PARP-1/2 inhibitor, with both strong catalytic inhibition and a PARP-trapping potential that is significantly greater than other PARP inhibitors. Catalytic inhibition causes cell death due to accumulation of irreparable DNA damage; talazoparib also traps PARP–DNA complexes, which may be more effective in cell death than enzymatic inhibition alone.
- **FDA Approval Date:** October 16, 2018
- **Indications:** Breast cancer, locally advanced or metastatic, BRCA mutated, HER2 negative

- **Dose:** 1 mg PO daily regardless of meals
- **Half-life:** 90 ± 58 hours
- **Metabolism:** Major P-glycoprotein/ABCB1 substrate; BCRP/ABCG2 substrate
- **Side Effects:** Fatigue, headache, alopecia, mild nausea/vomiting, diarrhea, anemia, neutropenia, thrombocytopenia, transaminitis, lymphopenia
- **Clinical Pearls:** Dose adjustment needed for creatinine clearance (CrCl) <60 mL/hr.

Taletrectinib

- **Alias:** DS-6051b; AB-106
- **Type Mechanism:** A selective ROS1/NTRK inhibitor that induces dramatic growth inhibition of both WT and G2032R-mutant ROS1-rearranged cancers or NTRK-rearranged cancers
- **Drug Class:** NTRK inhibitor
- **Phase:** Phase 1/2
- **Indications:** Neuroendocrine tumors or tumors harboring ROS1/NTRK rearrangements or patients with crizotinib-refractory ROS1+ NSCLC; phase 2 for NTRK fusion–driven solid tumors
- **Dose:** RP2D: 800 mg PO daily
- **Side Effects:** Nausea/vomiting, diarrhea

(Papadopoulos et al., 2020)

Tamoxifen

- **Brand Name:** Soltamox
- **Type Mechanism:** Selective estrogen receptor modulator
- **Drug Class:** Anti-estrogen
- **FDA Approval Date:** 1977
- **Indications:** Metastatic breast cancer, adjuvant treatment of early-stage breast cancer, DCIS, reduction of breast cancer incidence in women at high risk
- **Dose:** 20 mg oral daily
- **Half-life:** 5–7 days
- **Metabolism:** CYP450 including CYP3A, CYP2D6, CYP2C9, CYP2C19, and CYP2B6
- **Side Effects:** Endometrial cancer, uterine carcinoma, thromboembolism, LFT abnormalities, cataracts, musculoskeletal pain, fatigue, vaginal dryness

Telaglenastat

- **Alias:** CB839
- **Type Mechanism:** An orally bioavailable inhibitor of glutaminase that selectively and irreversibly inhibits glutaminase, a mitochondrial enzyme that is essential for the conversion of the amino acid glutamine into glutamate. By blocking glutamine utilization, proliferation in

rapidly growing cells is impaired. Glutamine-dependent tumors rely on the conversion of exogenous glutamine into glutamate and glutamate metabolites to both provide energy and generate building blocks.

- **Drug Class:** Glutaminase inhibitor
- **Indications:** NRF2-mutated, nonsquamous NSCLC; metastatic/refractory RAS WT CRC; advanced MDS; phase 2 in combination with cabozantinib and telaglenastat failed to meet primary end point in RCC
- **Dose:** 800 mg PO BID
- **Half-life:** 2 to 4 hours
- **Side Effects:** Fatigue, nausea, ALT/AST increase, photophobia, vomiting, ALP increase, decreased appetite

(Harding et al., 2021)

Temsirolimus

- **Alias:** CCI-779
- **Brand Name:** Torisel
- **Type Mechanism:** An ester analog of rapamycin that binds to and inhibits mTOR, resulting in a reduced expression of mRNAs necessary for cell-cycle progression and arresting cells in the G1 phase of the cell cycle
- **FDA Approval Date:** May 30, 2007
- **Indications:** RCC
- **Dose:** 25 mg infusion over 30 to 60 minutes once a week. Pretreatment with antihistamine recommended.
- **Half-life:** 17.3 hours
- **Metabolism:** Major CYP3A4 substrate
- **Side Effects:** Rash, asthenia, mucositis, nausea, edema, anorexia, anemia, hyperglycemia, hyperlipidemia
- **Clinical Pearls:** For management of fatigue: Encourage exercise and good sleep hygiene, initiate oral care early on (soft toothbrush, salt, and soda swish), avoid direct sunlight, use moisturizers after bathing, use mild soap for bathing, antihistamines for itching, be aware of possibility of lung toxicity, monitor fasting triglycerides and cholesterol. Levels may increase while on treatment.

Tepotinib

- **Alias:** MSC2156119J; EMD1214063
- **Brand Name:** Tepmetko
- **Type Mechanism:** An oral highly selective MET inhibitor that inhibits MET phosphorylation and downstream signaling
- **FDA Approval Date:** February 3, 2021
- **Indications:** FDA approved for metastatic NSCLC with MET alterations

- **Dose:** 500 mg PO daily 30 minutes after breakfast
- **Half-life:** 46 hours
- **Side Effects:** Peripheral edema, increased lipase/amylase, nausea, diarrhea, blood creatinine increased

(Falchook et al., 2020; Paik et al., 2020)

Tivantinib

- **Alias:** ARQ 197
- **Type Mechanism:** An orally bioavailable small molecule that binds to the MET protein and disrupts MET signal transduction pathways
- **Phase:** Phase 2/3
- **Indications:** HCC and in phase 2 clinical trials with many cancer types, including NSCLC, prostate, breast, and H&N
- **Dose:** 240 to 360 mg PO BID
- **Half-life:** 2 hours
- **Side Effects:** Fatigue, nausea, neutropenia, anemia, asthenia

(Rosen et al., 2011; Yap et al., 2011)

Toripalimab

- **Alias:** TAB001
- **Type Mechanism:** A humanized IgG4 mAb directed against the negative immunoregulatory human cell-surface

receptor PD-1. It binds to PD-1 and inhibits the binding of PD-1 to its ligands, PD-L1 and PD-L2. This prevents the activation of PD-1 and its downstream signaling pathways. This may restore immune function through the activation of both T cells and T-cell–mediated immune responses against tumor cells.
- **Drug Class:** Anti–PD-1 mAb
- **Phase:** Phase 2/3
- **Indications:** Neoadjuvant treatment in resectable stage 3 NSCLC, advanced melanoma
- **Dose:** 3 or 10 mg/kg IV days 1 and 15 of 28 days or flat dose of 240 or 360 mg IV day 1 of a 21-day cycle
- **Half-life:** 7.7 to 14 days
- **Side Effects:** Peripheral neuropathy, leukopenia, anemia, neutropenia, ALT/AST elevations, nausea, decreased appetite, thrombocytopenia, asthenia, maculopapular rash, pneumonitis

(Tang et al., 2020)

Trametinib

- **Alias:** GSK1120212; JTP-74057
- **Brand Name:** Mekinist
- **Type Mechanism:** An orally bioavailable molecule that specifically binds to and inhibits MEK1/2
- **FDA Approval Date:** May 29, 2013

- **Indications:**
  - FDA approved for (1) BRAF V600E– or V600K-mutated metastatic melanoma, and (2) in combination with dabrafenib for BRAF V600E– mutated metastatic NSCLC
    - First FDA-approved MEK inhibitor
- **Dose:** 2 mg PO daily
- **Half-life:** 4 to 5 days
- **Metabolism:** Weak CYP2C8 inhibitor and weak/moderate CYP3A4 inducer
- **Side Effects:** Rash or dermatitis acneiform, diarrhea, peripheral edema, fatigue, HTN, transaminitis
- **Clinical Pearls:** To prevent rash, avoid sun exposure and harsh soaps. Encourage patients to avoid spicy and acidic foods. Remain hydrated. Encourage antidiarrheal and antacid medication. Instruct patients to report visual changes immediately. Obtain baseline retinal and retinal vein examination.

Trastuzumab

- **Alias:** Biosimilar ABP 980; biosimilar PF-05280014
- **Brand Name:** Herceptin
- **Type Mechanism:** A recombinant humanized mAb directed against the HER2, inducing an ADCC against tumor cells that overexpress HER2
- **FDA Approval Date:** September 25, 1998
- **Indications:** FDA approved for the treatment of HER2-overexpressing breast cancer in adjuvant or metastatic setting and HER2-overexpressing gastric cancer
- **Dose:** Adjuvant or metastatic breast: Initial dose of 4 mg/kg over 90-minute IV infusion followed by subsequent weekly doses of 2 mg/kg as 30-minute IV infusion. Metastatic gastric: Initial dose of 8 mg/kg over 90-minute IV infusion followed by 6 mg/kg over 30- to 90-minute IV infusion Q 3 weeks
- **Half-life:** 2 days (for doses <10 mg)
- **Metabolism:** Cardiomyopathy, infusion reactions, embryo–fetal toxicity, and pulmonary toxicity (U.S. box warning); headache; diarrhea; nausea; chills; neutropenia
- **Side Effects:** Infusion reaction common— observe closely during loading dose; LVEF should be evaluated in patients before starting therapy and monitored Q 2 months.

Trastuzumab deruxtecan-nxki

- **Brand Name:** Enhertu
- **Drug Class:** Antibody–drug conjugate
- **Mechanism of Action:** HER2 antibody– drug conjugate that incorporates the

HER2-targeted actions of trastuzumab with topoisomerase–inhibitor conjugate. Composed of a humanized anti-HER2 IgG1 covalently linked to topoisomerase inhibitor, DXd, and exatecan derivative

- **FDA Approval Date:** December 20, 2019
- **Indications:** Patients with unresectable or metastatic HER2-positive breast cancer who have received two or more prior anti-HER2-based regimens in the metastatic setting
- **Dose:** 5.4 mg/kg IV infusion every 3 weeks
- **Half-life:** Median 5.5–5.8 days
- **Metabolism:** Primarily metabolized by CYP3A4. Low potential to inhibit OAT1/3, OCT1/2, P-gp, BCRP
- **Side Effects:** Nausea/vomiting, diarrhea, decreased appetite, interstitial lung disease, neutropenia, thrombocytopenia, LV dysfunction, hypokalemia, alopecia, headache

Tremelimumab

- **Alias:** CP-675,206; CP-675; anti-CTLA4 human mAb CP-675,206
- **Type Mechanism:** A human IgG2 mAb directed against the human TCR protein CTLA4 that binds to CTLA4 on activated T lymphocytes and blocks the binding of the APC ligands B7-1 (CD80) and B7-2 (CD86) to CTLA4, resulting in the inhibition of CTLA4-mediated downregulation of T-cell activation
- **Phase:** Phase 2
- **Indications:** Advanced HCC or biliary tract cancer, TNBC, germ cell tumor, esophageal cancer, urothelial carcinoma (phase 3 global study), high-risk STS, and NSCLC
- **Dose:** 1 mg/kg IV Q 4 weeks for 6 doses, then Q 12 weeks for 3 doses
- **Half-life:** 22 days
- **Side Effects:** Diarrhea, colitis, fatigue, nausea, skin rash, hypophysitis, pruritus

(Comin-Anduix et al., 2016)

Tucatinib

- **Alias:** ARRY380; irbinitinib; ONT-380
- **Brand Name:** Tukysa
- **Type Mechanism:** A TKI that is highly selective for the HER2 kinase domain, with minimal inhibition of EGFR. It inhibits HER2 and HER3 phosphorylation, resulting in downstream inhibition of MAPK and AKT signaling and cell proliferation; tucatinib demonstrated antitumor activity in HER2-expressing tumor cells and inhibited the growth of HER2-expressing tumors.
- **Drug Class:** HER2 TKI

- **FDA Approval Date:** April 17, 2020
- **Indications:** Advanced, unresectable, or metastatic HER2-positive breast cancer
- **Dose:** 300 mg PO BID (in combination with trastuzumab and capecitabine)
- **Half-life:** ~8.5 hours
- **Metabolism:** Major CYP2C8; minor CYP3A4; major CYP3A4; P-glycoprotein/ABCB1 inhibitors
- **Side Effects:** Palmar–plantar erythrodysesthesia, skin rash, hypomagnesemia, hypophosphatemia, weight loss, loss of appetite, diarrhea, nausea, stomatitis, vomiting, anemia, ALT/AST elevations, hyperbilirubinemia, peripheral neuropathy, headache, fatigue

Uprosertib

- **Alias:** GSK2141795
- **Type Mechanism:** Akt inhibitor GSK2141795 binds to and inhibits the activity of Akt, which may result in inhibition of the PI3K/Akt signaling pathway and tumor cell proliferation and the induction of tumor cell apoptosis. Activation of the PI3K/Akt signaling pathway is frequently associated with tumorigenesis, and dysregulated PI3K/Akt signaling may contribute to tumor resistance to a variety of antineoplastic agents.
- **Drug Class:** AKT inhibitor
- **Phase:** Phase 1
- **Indications:** TNBC or BRAF WT advanced melanoma (phase 1 study terminated); relapsed/refractory cervical cancer (phase 2 trial terminated); MUM
- **Dose:** 25 to 50 mg PO daily (in combination with trametinib)
- **Side Effects:** Diarrhea, rash, mucositis, colitis
- **Clinical Pearls:** Phase 1 study terminated early owing to futility in continuous dosing and intermittent dosing.

(Tolcher et al., 2020)

Urelumab

- **Alias:** BMS-663513; anti-4-1BB mAb
- **Type Mechanism:** A humanized agonistic mAb targeting the CD137 receptor with potential immunostimulatory and antineoplastic activities. Urelumab specifically binds to and activates CD137-expressing immune cells, stimulating an immune response, in particular a cytotoxic T-cell response, against tumor cells.
- **Drug Class:** Anti-4-1BB/CD137 mAb
- **Phase:** Phase 1/2
- **Indications:** Stages I to 2B pancreatic cancer before and after surgery; PD-L1–negative melanoma; NSCLC after failing PD-1/PD-L1 therapy

- **Dose:** 0.1 mg/kg IV Q 3 weeks
- **Half-life:** ~18 days
- **Side Effects:** Nausea, fatigue, ALT/ AST elevations, rash, pruritus, decreased appetite, pyrexia, diarrhea, leukopenia, thrombocytopenia, asthenia

(Segal et al., 2017)

Vandetanib

- **Alias:** AZD6474; ZD6474; Zactima; Zictifa
- **Brand Name:** Caprelsa
- **Type Mechanism:** A multikinase inhibitor including EGFR, VEGF, RET, protein tyrosine kinase 6, TIE-2, EPH kinase receptors, and SRC kinase receptors, selectively blocking intracellular signaling, angiogenesis, and cellular proliferation
- **Drug Class:** Multikinase inhibitor
- **FDA Approval Date:** April 6, 2011
- **Indications:** Locally advanced or metastatic MTC
- **Dose:** 300 mg PO daily
- **Metabolism:** Major CYP3A4 substrate
- **Side Effects:** QT prolongation, HTN, acneiform rash, pruritus, skin rash, xeroderma, hypocalcemia, abdominal pain, diarrhea, colitis, headache, fatigue, ALT elevation

Vanucizumab

- **Alias:** RG7221; RO5520985
- **Type Mechanism:** An antiangiogenic, first-in-class, bispecific mAb targeting VEGF-A and ANG-2
- **Phase:** Phase 2
- **Indications:** With FOLFOX versus FOLFOX + bevacizumab in untreated, mCRC
- **Dose:** 2,000 mg IV Q 2 weeks in combination with chemotherapy
- **Half-life:** 6 to 9 days
- **Side Effects:** HTN, asthenia, headache, hemorrhage, thrombosis

(Hidalgo et al., 2018)

Veliparib

- **Alias:** ABT-888
- **Type Mechanism:** A PARP-1 and PARP-2 inhibitor with chemosensitizing and antitumor activities. With no antiproliferative effects as a single agent at therapeutic concentrations, ABT-888 inhibits PARPs, thereby inhibiting DNA repair and potentiating the cytotoxicity of DNA-damaging agents.
- **Drug Class:** PARP inhibitor
- **Phase:** Phase 3

- **Indications:** Advanced squamous cell lung cancer; locally, advanced unresectable BRCA-associated breast cancer; high-grade serous epithelial ovarian, fallopian, or primary peritoneal carcinoma with BRCA mutation
- **Dose:** 120 to 150 mg PO BID for 7 days or 5 days on, 2 days off, or continuously (in combination with paclitaxel and carboplatin), then continue as maintenance at dose of 300 to 400 mg PO BID (without chemotherapy)
- **Half-life:** 5.18 hours
- **Side Effects:** Nausea, vomiting, fatigue, anemia, thrombocytopenia, neutropenia, diarrhea, leukopenia, loss of appetite

(Gojo et al., 2017; Isakoff et al., 2016)

Vemurafenib

- **Alias:** RO5185426; PLX4032; RG7204
- **Brand Name:** Zelboraf
- **Type Mechanism:** A PARP-1 and PARP-2 inhibitor with chemosensitizing and antitumor activities. With no antiproliferative effects as a single agent at therapeutic concentrations, ABT-888 inhibits PARPs, thereby inhibiting DNA repair and potentiating the cytotoxicity of DNA-damaging agents.

- **Drug Class:** BRAF kinase inhibitor
- **FDA Approval Date:** August 17, 2011
- **Indications:** Unresectable, metastatic melanoma; Erdheim–Chester disease with BRAF V600 mutation
- **Dose:** 960 mg PO Q 12 hours
- **Half-life:** 57 hours
- **Metabolism:** Major CYP3A4 substrate
- **Side Effects:** Prolonged QT, HTN, peripheral edema, headache, skin rash, neuropathy, fatigue, palmar–plantar erythrodysesthesia, nausea, vomiting, decreased appetite, diarrhea, cutaneous papilloma, SCC of skin, myalgia/arthralgia, increased GGT

Venetoclax

- **Alias:** ABT 199; GDC-0199; RG7601; SureCN523816; UN2-N54AIC43PW
- **Type Mechanism:** An orally bioavailable, selective small-molecule inhibitor of the antiapoptotic protein BCL-2
- **FDA Approval Date:** April 11, 2016
- **Indications:** FDA approved in April 2016 for patients with CLL who have 17p deletion chromosome
- **Dose:** Escalation weekly up to 400 mg PO daily. Give on a fasting stomach (food will increase bioavailability of drug). Dose escalation to gradually debulk and reduce the risk of TLS.

Consider antihyperuricemic therapy and hydration based on tumor lysis risk.
- **Half-life:** 26 hours
- **Side Effects:** Peripheral edema, nausea/diarrhea, fatigue, upper respiratory tract infection, cough, TLS, neutropenia, thrombocytopenia

Vistusertib

- **Alias:** AZD2014
- **Type Mechanism:** An inhibitor of the mTOR that inhibits the activity of mTOR, which may result in the induction of tumor cell apoptosis and a decrease in tumor cell proliferation
- **Drug Class:** mTOR kinase inhibitor
- **Phase:** Phase 2
- **Indications:** Phase 2 in metastatic ovarian cancer and NSCLC shows promise. November 2018, Astra Zeneca drops vistusertib owing to the lack of efficacy and toxicity. December 2019, Vistusertib was shown to be less effective in combination with fulvestrant than everolimus and fulvestrant.

(Schmid et al., 2019)

Vopratelimab

- **Alias:** JTX-2011
- **Type Mechanism:** An agonist mAb that specifically binds to the inducible CO-stimulator of T cells (ICOS) to generate an antitumor immune response. ICOS, a T-cell–specific, CD28 superfamily costimulatory molecule and immune checkpoint protein, is normally expressed on certain activated T cells and plays a key role in the proliferation and activation of T cells.
- **Drug Class:** ICOS mAb
- **Phase:** Phase 2
- **Indications:** NSCLC with TISvopra predictive biomarker; urothelial cancer
- **Dose:** 0.03 to 0.1 mg/kg IV Q 3 weeks (usually in combination with ipilimumab 3 mg/kg IV for 4 doses or nivolumab 240 mg IV Q 3 weeks)
- **Side Effects:** Anemia, hypoxia, diarrhea, infusion reactions with chills, pyrexia, neck pain, dizziness, nausea (can be delayed up to 6 hours post infusion)

(Martinez-Cannon et al., 2017)

Vorinostat

- **Alias:** MK 0683; SAHA
- **Brand Name:** Zolinza
- **Type Mechanism:** An orally available, synthetic hydroxamic acid derivative that binds to the catalytic domain of the HDACs, allowing the hydroxamic moiety to chelate zinc ion, thereby inhibiting deacetylation

and leading to an accumulation of both hyperacetylated histones and transcription factors
- **FDA Approval Date:** October 6, 2006
- **Indications:** CTCL that is progressive, persistent, or recurrent after two lines of treatment
- **Dose:** 400 mg PO daily with food. Take with plenty of water and keep hydrated.
- **Half-life:** 2 hours
- **Side Effects:** Fatigue, peripheral edema, alopecia, nausea/diarrhea, pruritus, hyperglycemia, proteinuria

Zanidatamab

- **Alias:** ZW25
- **Type Mechanism:** An engineered IgG1 bispecific mAb that targets two different nonoverlapping epitopes of the human TAA HER2, ECD2 and ECD4 resulting in dual HER2 signal blockade, HER2 clustering, and receptor internalization and downregulation. This also induces a CTL response and ADCC against tumor cells that overexpress HER2.
- **Drug Class:** Bispecific mAb
- **Phase:** Phase 3
- **Indications:** HER2-positive, metastatic breast cancer; first-line HER2-positive GE adenocarcinoma, HER2-amplified advanced, metastatic biliary tract cancer including cholangiocarcinoma and gallbladder cancer
- **Dose:** Three dosing schema are being studied: (1) 30 mg/kg IV Q 3 weeks, (2) 20 mg/kg IV Q 2 weeks, and (3) 1,200/1,600 mg IV Q 2 weeks.
- **Side Effects:** Diarrhea, infusion-related side effects (chills, fevers), fatigue, nausea/vomiting, dysgeusia, loss of appetite, peripheral neuropathy
- **Clinical Pearls:** Infusions should be premedicated with acetaminophen and diphenhydramine and given over 2 hours.

(Ku et al., 2021)

Ziv-Aflibercept

- **Brand Name:** Zaltrap
- **Type Mechanism:** Fusion protein inhibitor of VEGF
- **FDA Approval Date:** August 3, 2012
- **Indications:** FDA approved for mCRC that is resistant to or has progressed following an oxaliplatin-containing regimen
- **Dose:** 4 mg/kg IV infusion over 1 hour Q 2 weeks in combination with FOLFIRI
- **Half-life:** 6 days
- **Side Effects:** Diarrhea, proteinuria, increased AST and ALT, stomatitis, fatigue,

HTN, weight reduced, decreased appetite, epistaxis, abdominal pain, dysphonia, increased SCr, headache; hematologic: leukopenia, neutropenia, thrombocytopenia

Zotatifin

- **Alias:** eFT226
- **Brand Name:** Zotatifin
- **Type Mechanism:** A selective inhibitor of the eukaryotic translation initiation factor 4A (eIF4A) by targeting and binding to eIF4A, and promotes eIF4A binding to mRNA with specific polypurine motifs within their 5′-untranslated region (5′-UTR), leading to the formation of a stable sequence-specific ternary complex with eIF4A and mRNA (eIF4A-zotatifin-mRNA). This results in the translational repression of key oncogenes and antiapoptotic proteins involved in tumor cell proliferation, survival, and metastasis, such as KRAS, Myc, myeloid cell leukemia-1 (Mcl-1), B-cell lymphoma 2 (Bcl-2), CDK4 and CDK6, cyclin D, FGFR1 and FGFR2, HER2 (ERBB2), and β-catenin.
- **Drug Class:** eIF4A inhibitor
- **Phase:** Phase 2
- **Indications:** KRAS-mutant NSCLC and breast cancer
- **Dose:** 0.07 mg/kg IV on days 1 and 8 of a 21-day cycle

Index